KETO
COOKBOOK
FOR BEGINNERS

50+ RECIPES FOR ALL MEALS

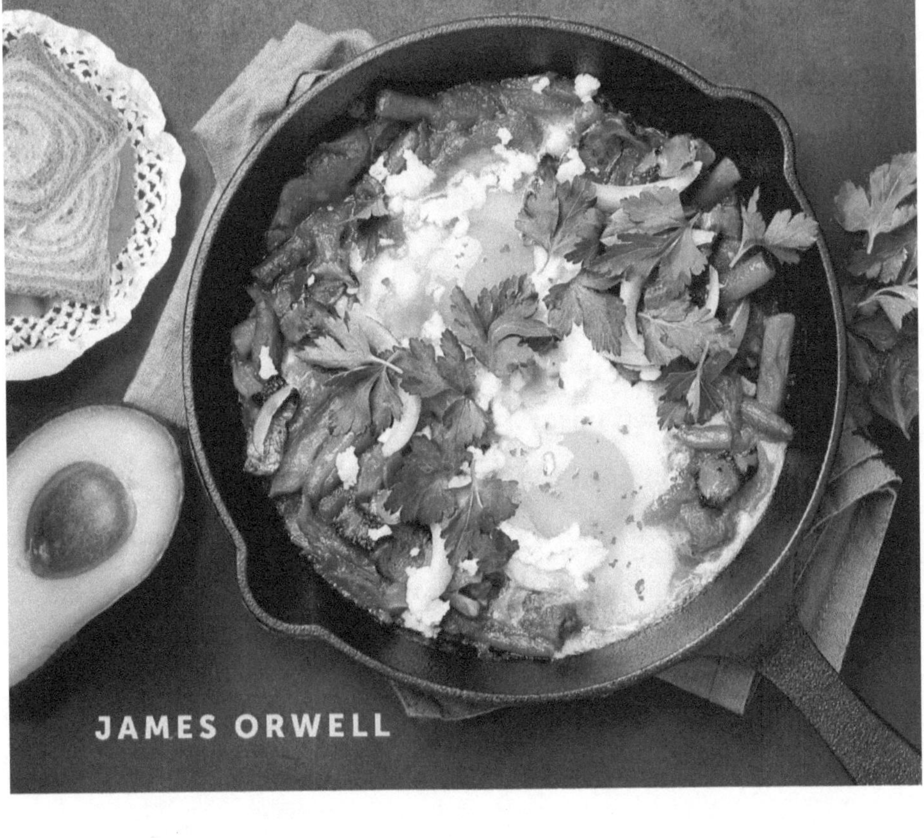

JAMES ORWELL

Table of Contents

BREAKFAST

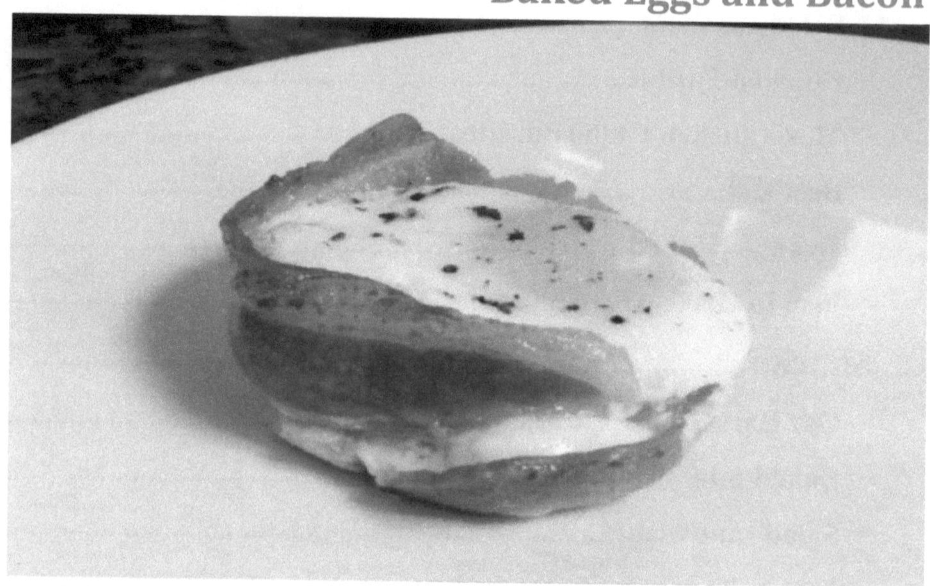

INGREDIENTS

6 slices bacon

6 eggs

1 non-stick muffin pan

INSTRUCTIONS

For each muffin cup, take one slice of bacon and wrap around 4 fingers to shape it into a circle.

Place in muffin cup.

Crack egg into the center.

Repeat for each serving.

Place muffin pan in oven and bake at 350 for about 40 minutes.

Cherry and Blueberry Smoothie

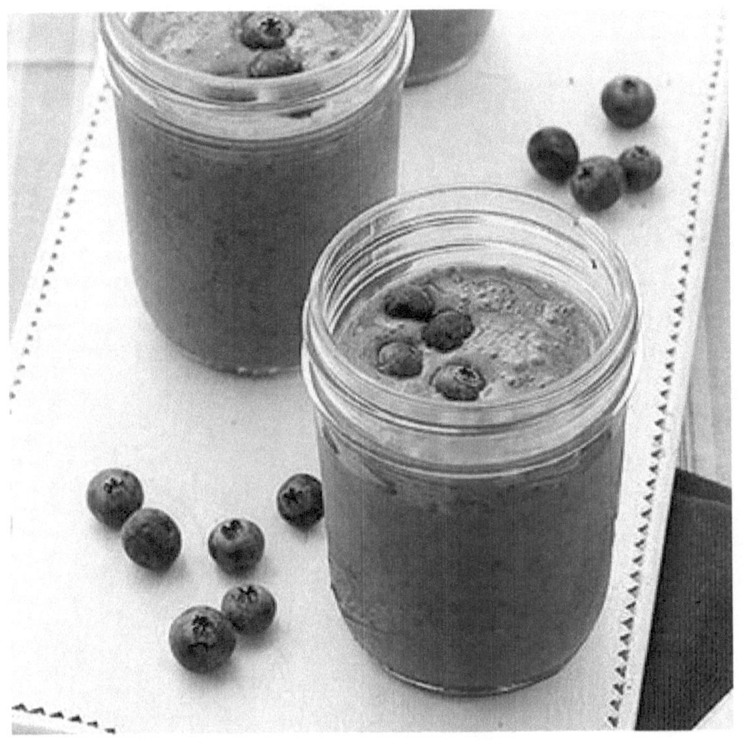

INGREDIENTS

4 ounces water

3/4 cup cherries, frozen

1 cup blueberries

3 scoops   protein powder , 21 grams of protien

4 1/2 teaspoons almonds, slivered

INSTRUCTIONS

If berries are fresh, rinse.

Blend ingredients until smooth

Pour into glass and enjoy

Chocolate Cherry Muffins

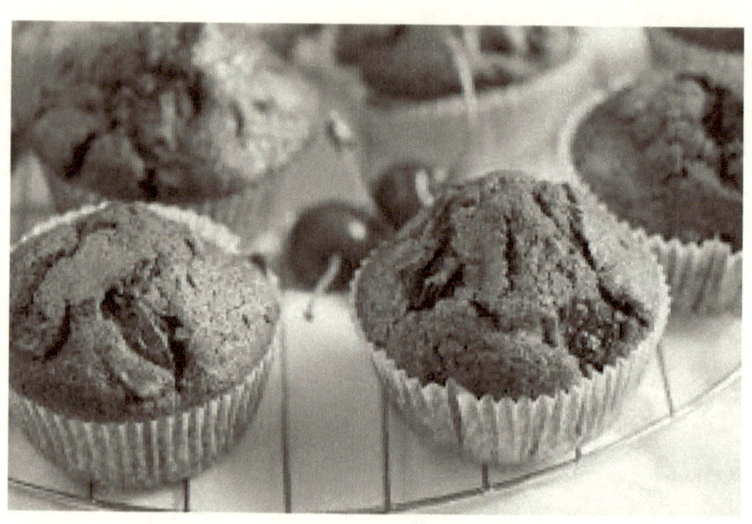

INGREDIENTS

Dry:

1 1/3 cups oat flour

4 (1 ounce) scoops chocolate flavored whey protein, (amount providing 84 grams protein), scant 1 cup

2 1/4 teaspoons pumpkin or apple pie spice

1 tablespoon non-aluminum baking powder

1 tablespoon grated orange rind, (optional)

Wet:

4 whole or 8 whites 4 whole eggs or 8 egg whites

Two tablespoons and two teaspoons fructose powder or syrup

2/3 cup applesauce

5 1/3 teaspoons canola oil

1 cup frozen pitted sweet cherries, coarsely chopped

INSTRUCTIONS

Preheat oven to 350 degrees F. Spray 12 muffin tins with non-stick spray and set aside. Sift dry ingredients into 1 1/2 quart mixing bowl, adding orange rind if desired. Stir; set aside. Combine all wet ingredients in blender except the cherries. Cover and process until smooth, stopping to scrape down sides. Or, whisk in mixing bowl. Add wet ingredients to dry ingredients. Stir until evenly mixed, scraping bottom of bowl to incorporate flour and remove lumps. Do not over-mix. Gently fold in cherries. Spoon batter into 12 muffin cups, evenly distributing it. Bake in preheated oven until firm to the touch, golden on top and around the edges, and a tooth pick inserted into the center comes out clean, about for 20 to 24 minutes. Allow to cool, then run a knife around edges to release muffins. Cover and refrigerate. Use within one week or freeze.

Variations

Divide batter between 16 muffin tins, filling any empty tins with water. Bake for 12 to 15 minutes or until muffins test done.

Breakfast Sundae

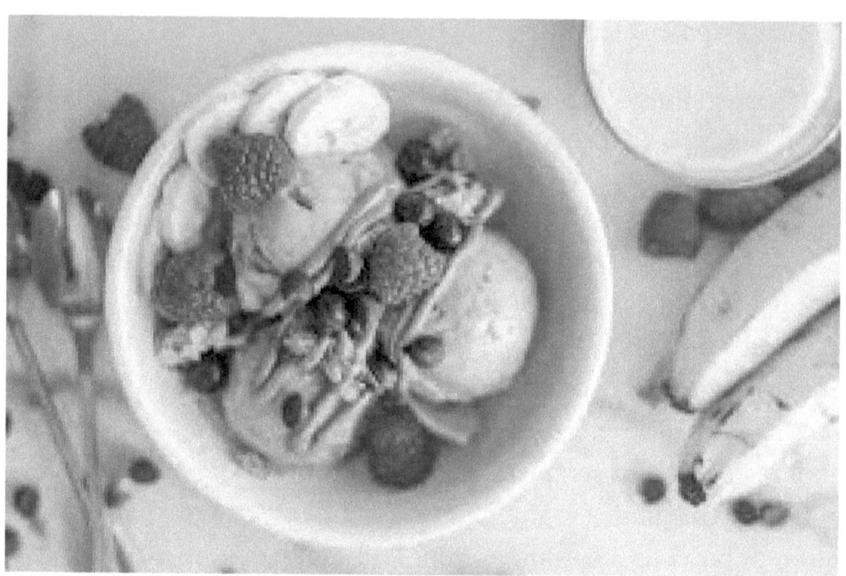

INGREDIENTS

1 cup low-fat cottage cheese

¾ teaspoon pure vanilla or maple extract, (non-alcohol, glycerine base)

1/8 teaspoon ground nutmeg or cinnamon

1 cup sliced strawberries

½ cup blueberries, fresh or frozen and thawed

1 fresh peach, pitted and sliced

8 cherries, pitted, fresh or frozen and thawed

12 almonds, toasted lightly, chopped coarsely, or 12 walnut or pecan halves, chopped coarsely

INSTRUCTIONS

Combine cottage cheese, vanilla or maple extract and spice in a medium-sized bowl. Arrange strawberries around the outer rim of a large cereal bowl or dinner plate. Use an ice cream scoop to shape cottage cheese and arrange on the plate. Top with blueberries, sliced peach and then cherries. Sprinkle nuts on top. (Feel free to double the amount of cherries. Just delete either the blueberries or peach.)

Crossfit Breakfast

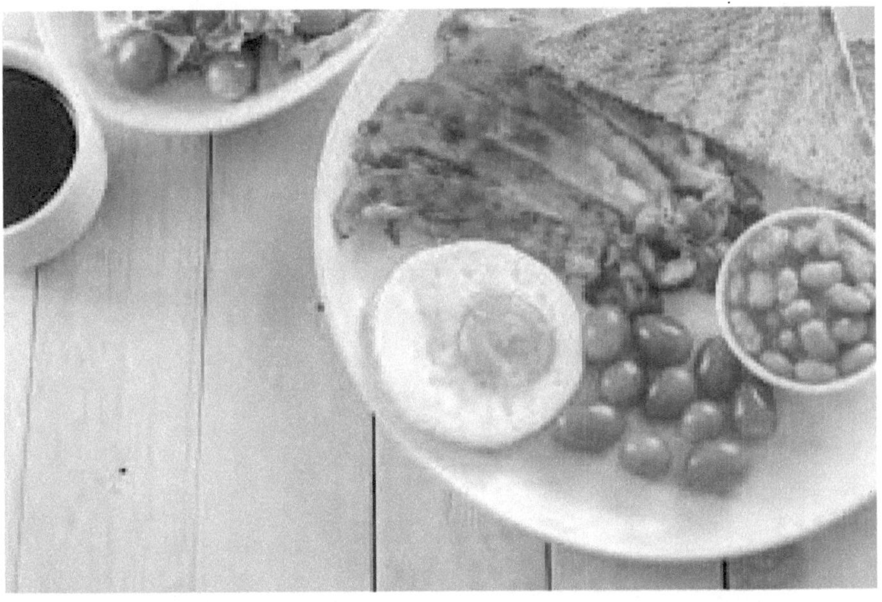

INGREDIENTS

1-6"   Low Carb tortilla or Pita

1/4cup rinsed black beans

1/4 cup salsa

1/2 cup diced tomatoes

1/4 cup diced orange pieces

1/2 cup egg substitute, scrambled w/ olive oil spray

1 ounce canadian bacon, seared and diced

1 ounce grated cheese

2 Tbsp. diced avocado

Cilantro to taste

INSTRUCTIONS

Place low carb tortilla or pita on plate and sprinkle with 1/2 ounce grated cheese, microwave on high 20 seconds. Cover with blackbeans & salsa. Place scrambled eggs on top. Sprinkle canadian bacon & 1/2 ounce cheese on top of that. Microwave on high 20 seconds. Add tomatoes, oranges and avocado. Sprinkle cilantro to taste.

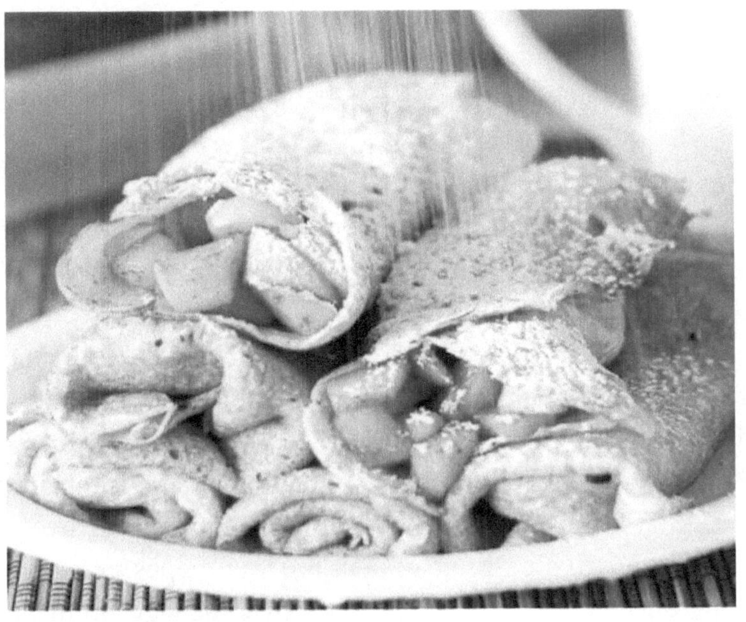

INGREDIENTS

2 whole eggs

6 ounces deli ham, diced fine

1/3 cup soy flour

1 cup 1-percent milk

1 red Delicious apples, peeled, cored and roughly chopped

2/3 cup unsweetened applesauce

2/3 cup cooked oatmeal

2 2/3 teaspoons olive oil

1/4 teaspoon cinnamon

INSTRUCTIONS

In a small mixing bowl, combine eggs, soy flour and milk to form a batter. This amount of batter will make four crepes. Pour 1/2 teaspoon oil into a nonstick saute pan or crepe pan. When the oil is hot, add a quarter of the batter to pan. Cover pan with another saute or crepe pan. Cook on medium-high heat until bottom is set and crepe will move easily in pan. To turn crepe over, securely place second pan over first and turn pan over. The crepe will then be in the second saute pan. The second side of the crepe should cook for only a minute or so to color it. Transfer crepe to serving plate and repeat process to make three more crepes. (If you need more oil in the crepe pan, omit oil from crepe filling and use it for cooking the crepes.) Place apples, applesauce, oatmeal, 2/3 teaspoon oil, ham and cinnamon in another saute pan to form crepe filling. Using low heat, cook mixture until apples are tender. When ready, divide filling amount the four crepes by placing it in a line along the center of each crepe. Fold over the sides to make a trifold. Serve immediately, two crepes per plate.

Mexican Omelet

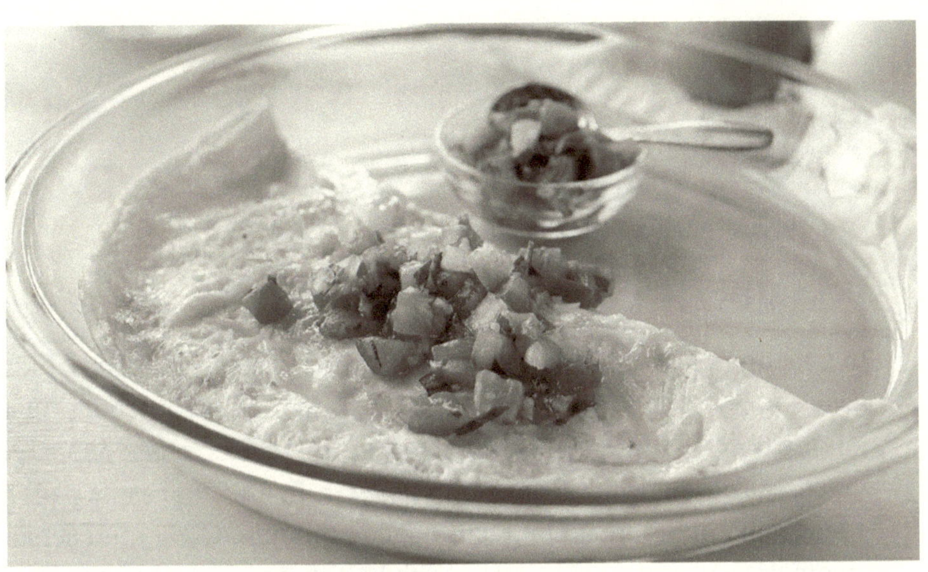

INGREDIENTS

2 large whole eggs

12 egg whites

3 cups onions, minced

½ cup cooked chickpeas

½ cup cooked kidney beans

1 cup green bell pepper, diced

1 cup red bell pepper, diced

2 cups mushrooms, minced

2 2/3 teaspoons olive oil, divided

1/8 teaspoon black pepper

1/8 teaspoon hot sauce, (or to taste)

1/8 teaspoon dry mustard

1/4 teaspoon turmeric

1/8 teaspoon chili powder

4 cloves garlic, minced, divided

INSTRUCTIONS

In a medium nonstick sauté pan, cook onion, garlic, chickpeas, kidney beans, peppers and mushrooms in 2/3 teaspoon oil until tender. In a mixing bowl, whip together whole eggs, egg whites, black pepper, hot sauce, mustard, turmeric, and chili powder. In a second sauté pan, heat 1 teaspoon oil before adding half the egg mixture. Cook until set and an omelet is formed. Fill omelet with half the vegetable mixture, fold over and serve. Repeat process to make second omelet.

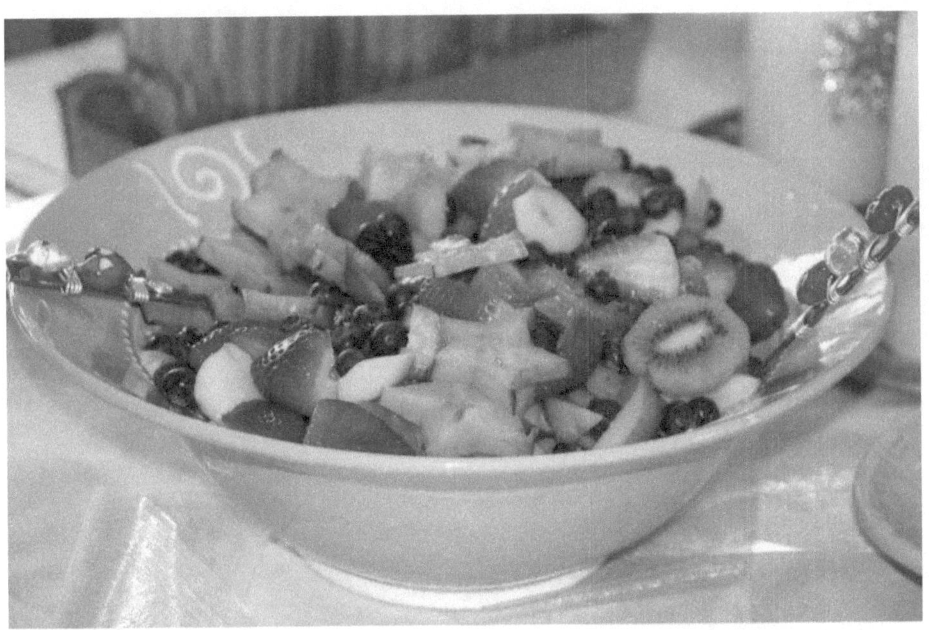

INGREDIENTS

3/4 cup low fat cottage cheese

1 cup fresh or reduced-sugar canned pineapple cubed

1/3 cup reduced-sugar canned mandarin oranges, drained

3 macadamia nuts, crushed

INSTRUCTIONS

Place cottage cheese in a bowl. Fold in pineapple, oranges, and nuts.

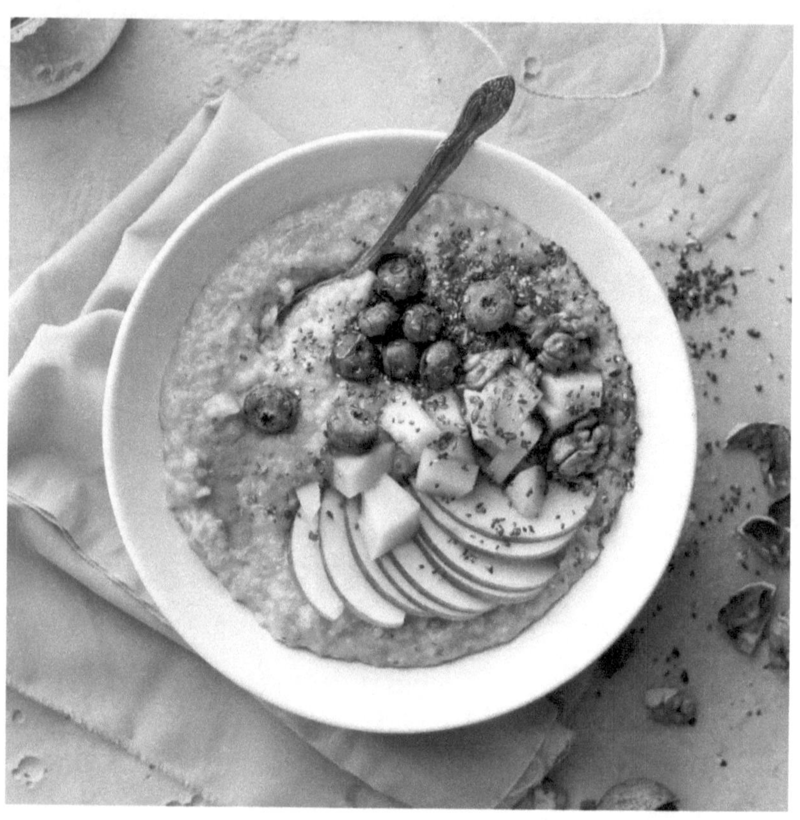

INGREDIENTS

1 cup cooked oatmeal

1/2 apple chopped

4 teaspoons natural peanut butter

Cinnamon to taste

1 cup lowfat cottage cheese

INSTRUCTIONS

Cook oatmeal. Mix in peanut butter, then the apple and then add cinnamon to taste.

Jellied Fruit Salad With Walnuts

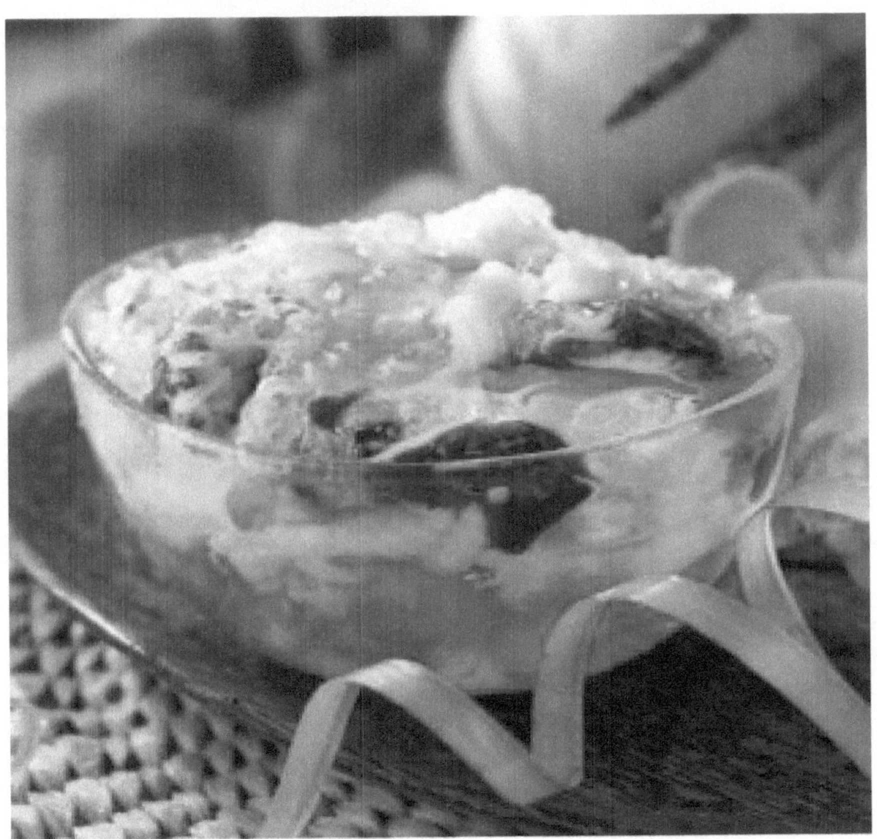

INGREDIENTS

4 envelopes Knox Unflavored Gelatin

1 kiwi fruit, peeled and diced

1 cup raspberries

1 cup strawberries, diced

1/2 cup seedless red grapes, halved

4 teaspoons walnuts, chopped

2 cups water

1 tablespoon banana extract

1 tablespoon orange extract

1/2 teaspoon strawberry extract

 Mint leaves

INSTRUCTIONS

In saucepan, place gelatin and water, stir until dissolved, then add fruit and extracts. Heat to a simmer, stirring gently for 10 minutes until the raspberries dissolve. Pour liquid into eight-inch by eight-inch by two inch pan and let cool. When Jellied Fruit Salad has set, place in four serving dishes and garnish with mint leaves.

Note: when choosing berries, look for those that are medium-sized and uniform in color. They should also feel solid to the touch and not be leaking juice.

LUNCH

Autumn Wild Rice

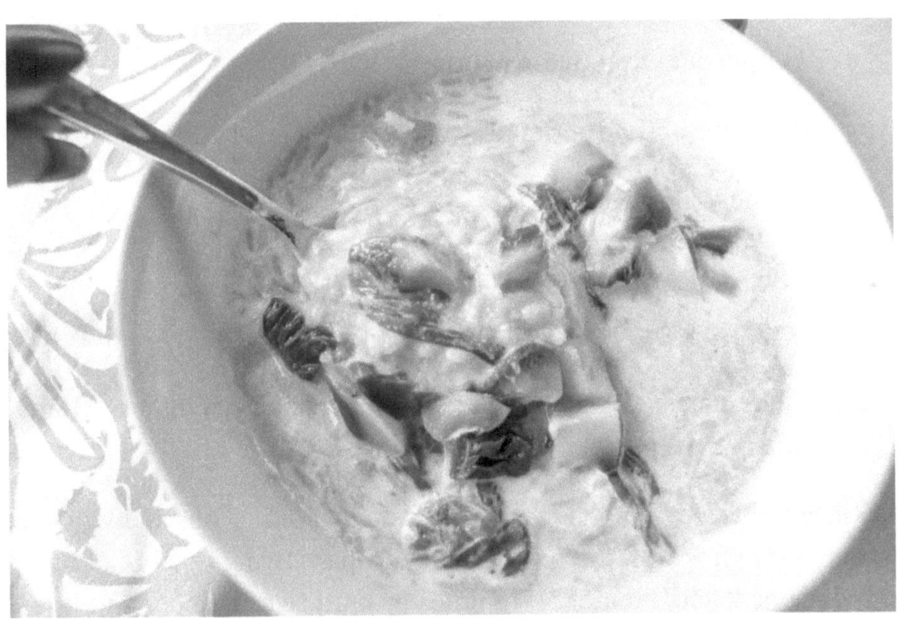

INGREDIENTS

2 tablespoons raisins

1/4 cup hot water

1/2 cup wild rice, uncooked

3 cups water, divided

2 cups apple, chopped

3/4 cup carrot, shredded

1/4 cup celery, chopped

1/4 cup green pepper, chopped

1-1/2 teaspoon chicken-flavored bouillon granules

1/4 teaspoon dried whole sage

1/8 teaspoon pepper

3/4 cup converted rice, uncooked

 fresh sage sprig, (optional)

 nonstick cooking spray

1 juice of 1 lemon

INSTRUCTIONS

Combine raisins and 1/4 cup hot water; let stand 5 minutes. Drain and set aside.

Rinse wild rice in 3 changes of hot water; drain. Combine wild rice and 1-1/2 cups water in a medium saucepan. Bring to a boil; cover, reduce heat and simmer 50 minutes or until rice is tender and liquid is absorbed. Remove pan from heat and set aside.

Coat a large nonstick skillet with cooking spray; place over a medium-high heat until hot. Add apple, carrot, celery and green pepper; sauté until crisp-tender. Remove skillet from heat and set aside.

Combine remaining 1-1/2 cups water, bouillon granules, sage and pepper in a large saucepan; bring to a boil. Stir in converted rice. Cover, reduce heat and simmer 20 minutes or until rice is tender and liquid is absorbed. Remove pan from heat; stir in reserved raisins, wild rice, apple mixture and juice of 1 lemon. Cover and let stand 5 minutes.

Transfer to a serving bowl. Garnish with a fresh sage sprig, if desired.

Curried Chicken Salaad with Grapes

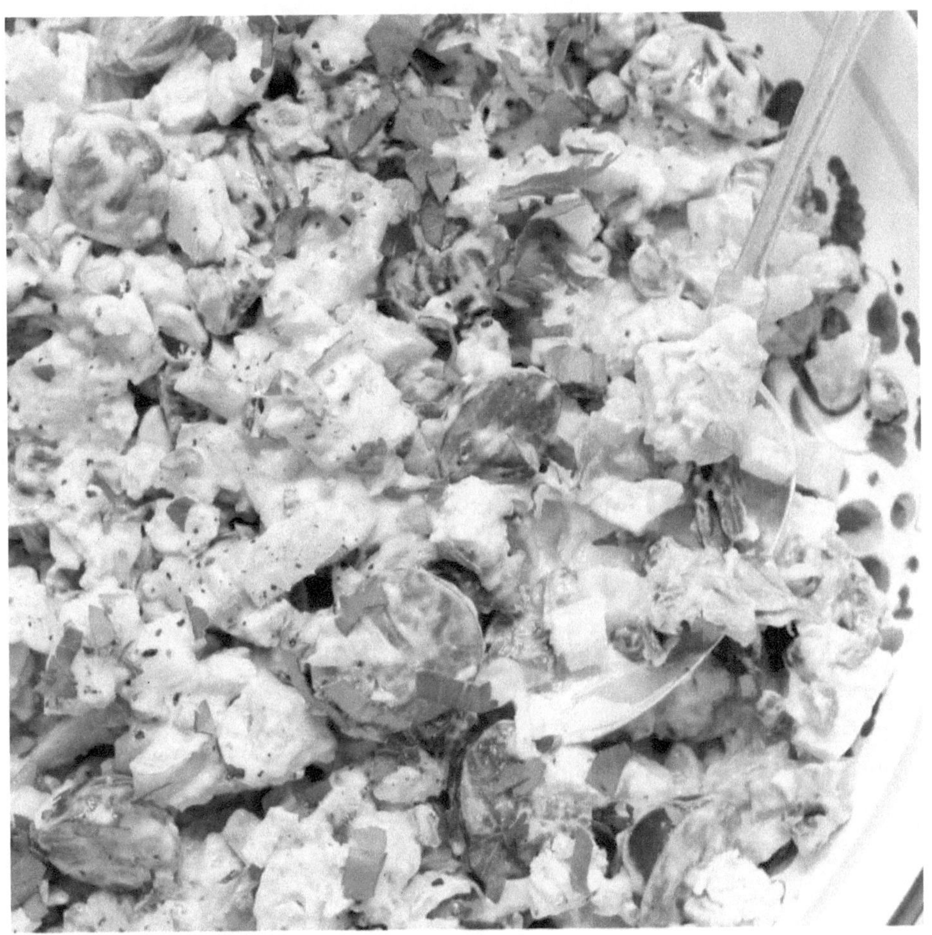

INGREDIENTS

1 lb. boneless, skinless chicken breasts

1/2 cup plain nonfat yogurt

1/4 cup mayonnaise, reduced fat

2 Tbsp. fresh lemon juice,, (about 1/2 lemon)

2 Tbsp. mango chutney, or apricot jam

2.5 tsp. curry powder, to taste

2 large celery stalks, finely diced

1 cup seedless red grapes, halved, or use chopped apple, mango or pineapple

1/4 cup pistachio nuts, shelled and unsalted, slivered almonds or coarsely chopped pecans will work too

INSTRUCTIONS

Trim any excess fat from the chicken. Place the chicken in a large skillet and add just enough water to cover it. Bring the water to a boil over high heat, reduce the heat to a simmer, cover and poach the chicken (steam it lightly in boiling water) for 7-10 minutes, until it is just cooked through (check by cutting into the thickest piece of chicken to make sure it is no longer pink). Rinse the chicken under cold water to cool it. Shred it by hand or chop it into 1/2-inch pieces.

Meanwhile, in a large bowl, combine the yogurt, mayonnaise, lemon juice, chutney or jam and curry powder. Stir in the chicken, celery, grapes, and nuts. Serve it immediately, or chill it for up to 48 hours.

Penne with Fresh Tomatoes and Basil

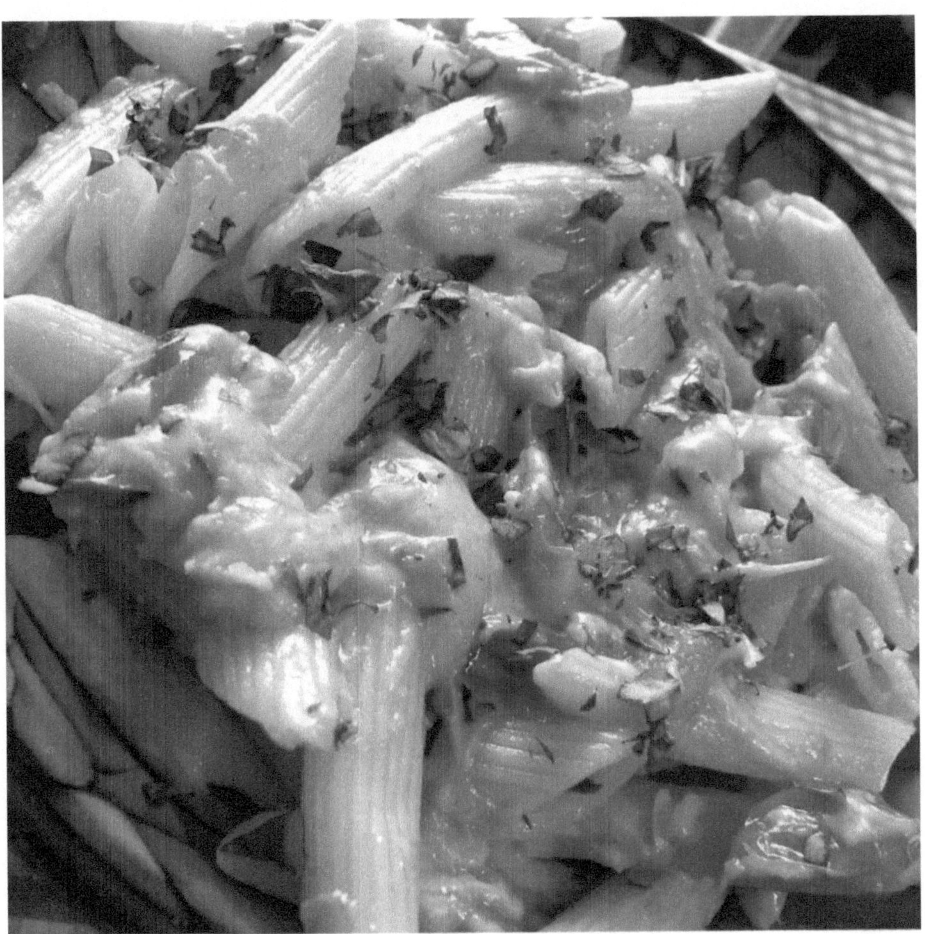

INGREDIENTS

1 pkg. penne or other cut pasta, 16 oz. package

2 lbs. fresh tomatoes, chopped about 8 tomatoes

1/3 cup olive oil, to taste

1 tsp. minced garlic, about 2 cloves

1/2 tsp. salt, to taste

20 leaves fresh basil, chopped

1/4 cup shredded Parmesan cheese, optional

INSTRUCTIONS

Cook the penne according to the package directions.

Meanwhile, in a large bowl, mix the tomatoes, oil, garlic, salt and basil. Smash the tomatoes in the oil with a fork or potato masher and let the mixture stand.

When the noodles are cooked, drain them well and toss them with the tomato mixture. Top it with Parmesan cheese, if desired.

Baby Spinach and Chickpea Salad

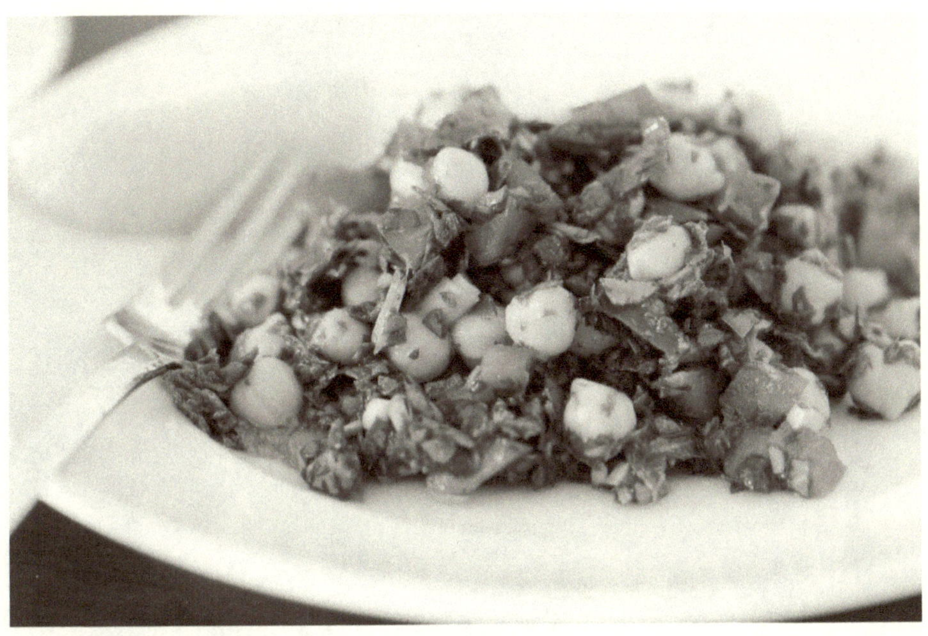

INGREDIENTS

1 1/2 cups   Chickpeas

1/2 medium red onion, half-moons, sliced thin

1 cup grape tomatoes, halved

Salt and pepper to taste

Balsamic vinegar, drizzle

1 tablespoon olive oil

INSTRUCTIONS

In a large bowl combine spinach, chickpeas, onion, and tomato. Add balsamic vinegar and olive oil. Season with salt and pepper. Toss to coat.

Barbecue Chicken Salad

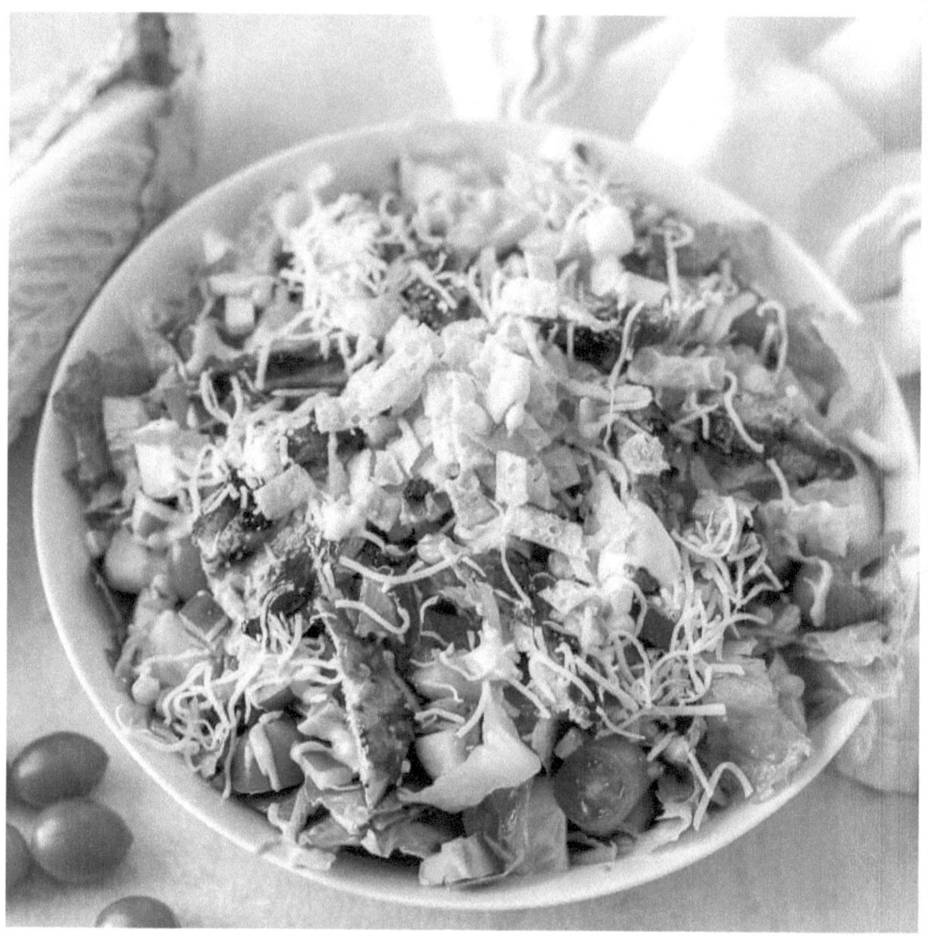

INGREDIENTS

4 ounces chicken tenderloin, diced (or skinless chicken breast)

2 cups bell pepper strips

1 1/2 cups onions, diced

1/2 cup Zoned Barbecue Sauce

3 cups garden salad mix, (lettuce and shredded red cabbage)

2 cups shredded cabbage, (or coleslaw mix)

1 1/3 teaspoons olive oil

1/8 teaspoon cider vinegar

1/8 teaspoon Worcestershire sauce

1 teaspoon minced garlic

  Salt and pepper to taste

INSTRUCTIONS

In a nonstick saute pan, add oil, chicken tenderloins, pepper, onion,
vinegar, Worcestershire sauce and garlic. Cook until chicken is
browned and vegetables are tender, then add Zoned Barbecue Sauce.
Cover and simmer for five minutes until mixture is hot, stirring
occasionally to blend flavors. Blend together garden salad mix and
shredded cabbage, then place blended salad-cabbage mixture on a
large oval plate. Spoon chicken and vegetable mixture into the center
of plate on top of salad-cabbage mixture. Sprinkle with salt and pepper
and serve immediately.

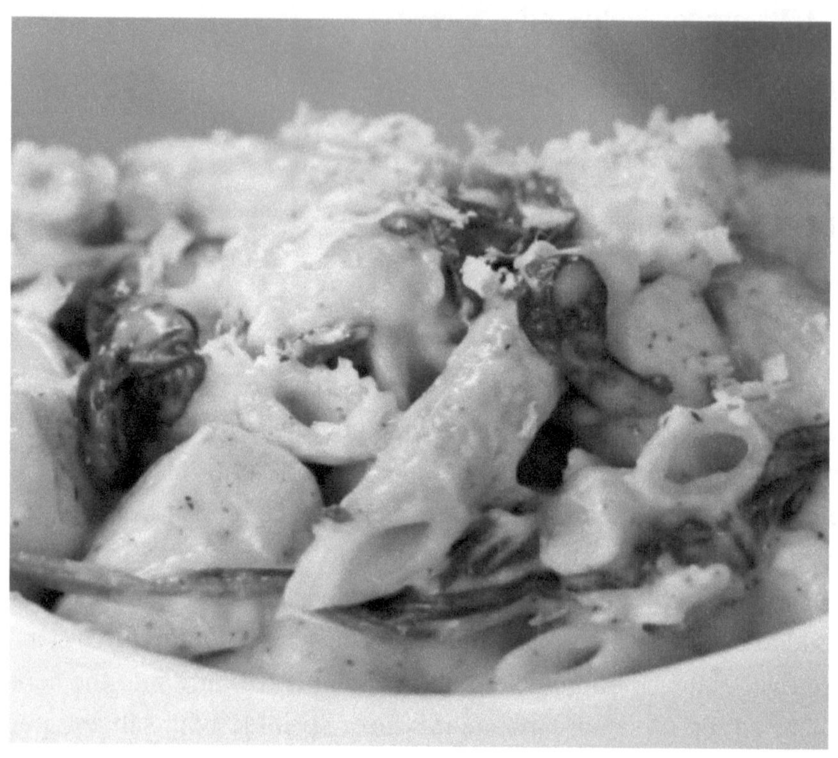

INGREDIENTS

3 cups whole wheat rotini

3 skinless, boneless chicken breast

1 T olive oil

¼ onion, chopped

1 cup fresh mushrooms, chopped

2 tablespoons Italian seasoning

½ tablespoon garlic powder

1 , (14.5 ounce) can low sodium tomato sauce

1 , (14.5 ounce) can low sodium diced tomatoes

Pepper to taste

2 tablespoons grated Low Sodium Parmesan cheese

INSTRUCTIONS

Bring a large pot of water to a boil. Add pasta and cook for 8 to 10 minutes or until al dente; drain and reserve. Cut chicken breast into small pieces about ½ inch in size. Place cut chicken in bowl and toss with 1T of olive oil.

In a large non-stick skillet over medium heat, cook chicken for about 15 and remove from pan. In same skillet over medium heat, combine onion, mushrooms, Italian seasoning, garlic powder, tomatoes with juice, tomato sauce and pepper; cook until onions are translucent. Add chicken to sauce remove from heat and add pasta. Sprinkle with Parmesan cheese on top.

Grilled Turkey Salad With Mandarin Oranges

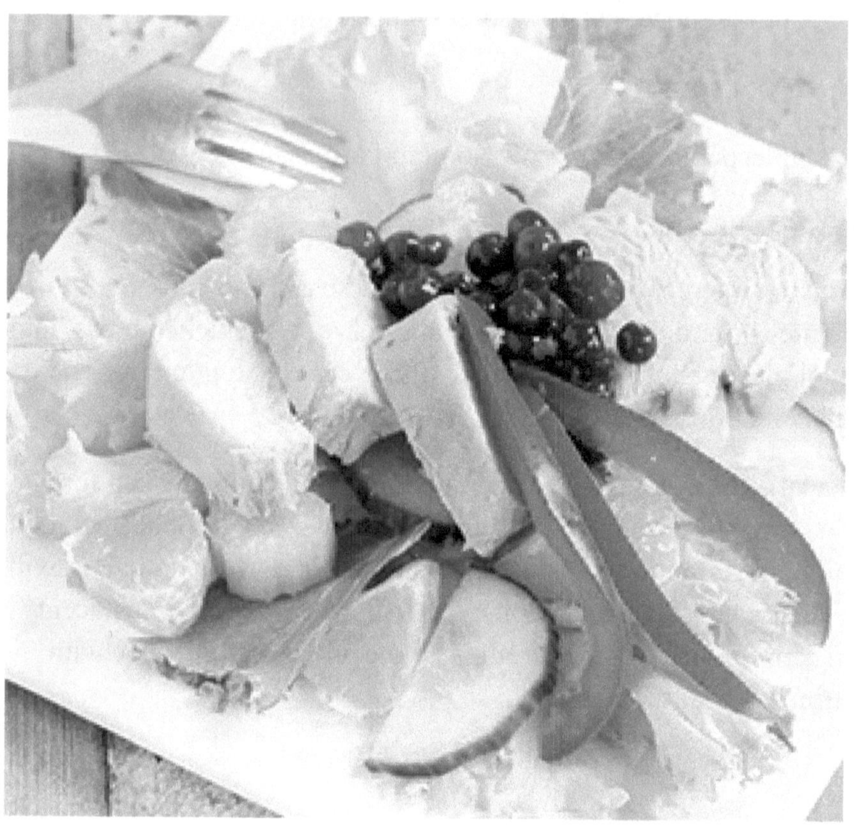

INGREDIENTS

4 ounces cooked turkey breast, cubed

1 cup celery, finely sliced

3/4 cup red onion, finely sliced

 Romaine lettuce

1/2 cup Zoned French Dressing, recipe to follow

1/3 cup unsweetened Mandarin oranges

1 peach

1 1/3 teaspoons olive oil

1/8 teaspoon turmeric

1 tablespoon fresh mint, chopped

INSTRUCTIONS

In a salad bowl, combine turkey, celery, onion, oil, Zoned French
Dressing, peach, oranges, tumeric and mint. Toss lightly to coat. On a
lunch plate place lettuce, top with turkey mixture and serve.

Greek Salad with Oregano Dressing

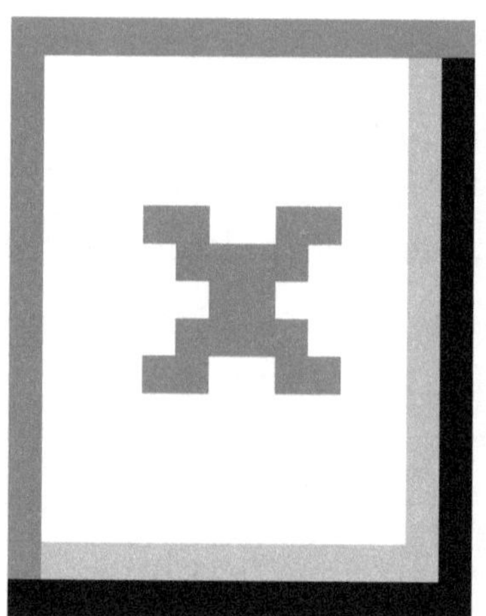

INGREDIENTS

5 cups loosely packed romaine lettuce, washed, patted dry, and torn into small pieces

1 cup canned artichoke hearts, drained and cut into bite-size pieces

2 medium tomatoes, cut into wedges

1 small red onion, thinly sliced

1/4 cup canned garbanzo beans, drained and rinsed 1 ounce feta cheese, crumbled

6 ounces extra-firm tofu, cut into 1/2-inch cubes

1 1/3 teaspoons extra-virgin olive oil

1 tablespoon red wine vinegar

2 tablespoons vegetable stock or water

1 small garlic clove, minced

1/4 teaspoon dried oregano, crumbled

1/4 teaspoon freshly ground black pepper

INSTRUCTIONS

Arrange lettuce on large dinner plate. Top with artichoke hearts, tomatoes, onions, garbanzo beans, feta cheese, and tofu.

In a small bowl, mix together olive oil, red wine vinegar, vegetable stock or water, garlic, oregano, and black pepper. Pour over salad and toss to evenly distribute dressing. Serve. Variation: If you have it on hand, try using cold baked or cold grilled tofu in this recipe. Many health food stores now carry prebaked or pre-grilled tofu in the refrigerator section.

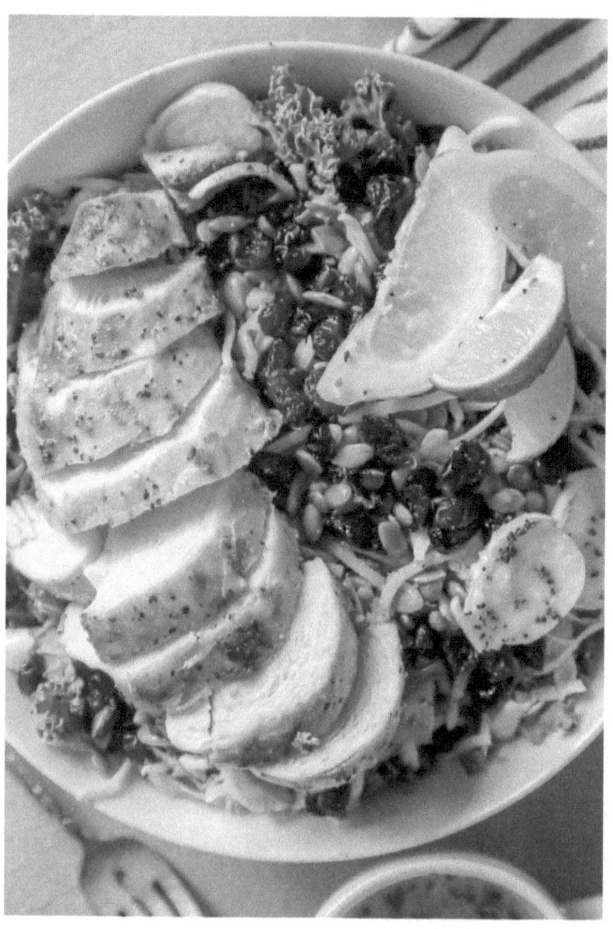

INGREDIENTS

2 c. chicken, cubed

2 c. celery, sliced

1 pkg. frozen green peas, (10 oz.)

1/2 c. almonds, slivered

2 tbsp. green pepper

1 tbsp. onion, grated

2 tbsp. pimento, diced

2 tbsp. lemon juice

1/2 tsp. salt

3/4 c. mayonnaise

1 c. grated American cheese

INSTRUCTIONS

Combine all ingredients thoroughly. Turn into buttered 2 quart casserole. Sprinkle with cheese and bake at 350 degrees for 25 minutes or until cheese is melted. Makes 10 servings and this can be frozen.

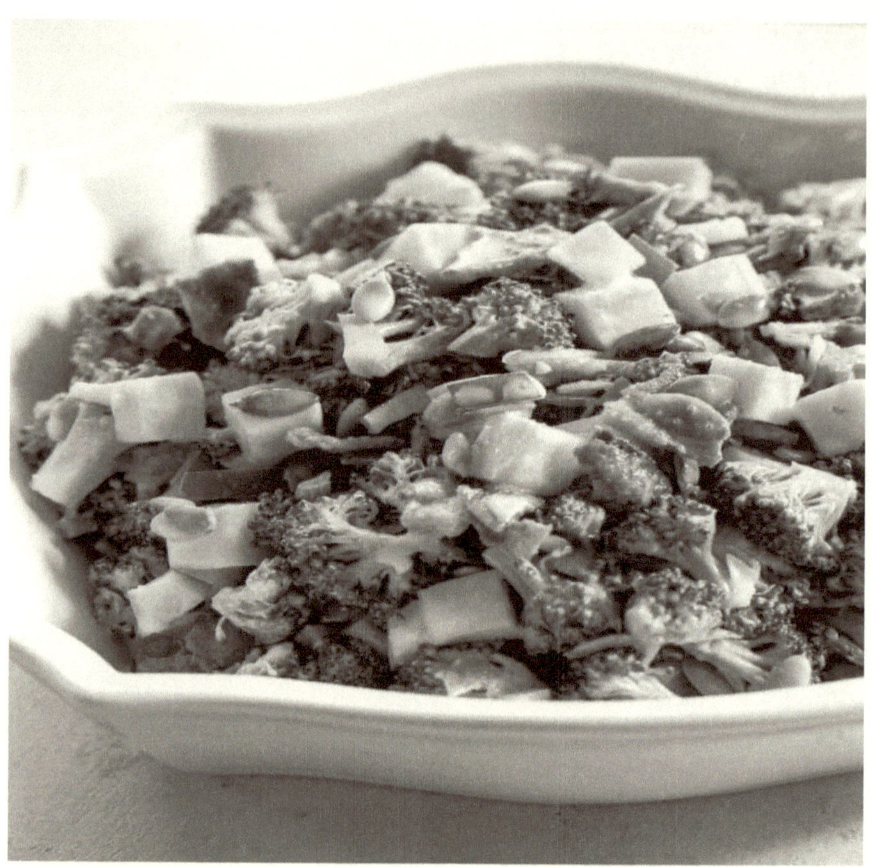

INGREDIENTS

FOR THE SALAD

kosher salt

3 heads broccoli, cut into bite-size pieces

1/2 c. shredded Cheddar

1/4 red onion, thinly sliced

1/4 c. toasted sliced almonds

3 slices bacon, cooked and crumbled

2 tbsp. freshly chopped chives

FOR THE DRESSING

2/3 c. mayonnaise

3 tbsp. apple cider vinegar

1 tbsp. dijon mustard

Kosher salt

Freshly ground black pepper

INSTRUCTIONS

In a medium pot or saucepan, bring 6 cups of salted water to a boil. While waiting for the water to boil, prepare a large bowl with ice water.

Add broccoli florets to the boiling water and cook until tender, 1 to 2 minutes. Remove with a slotted spoon and place in the prepared bowl of ice water. When cool, drain florets in a colander.

In a medium bowl, whisk to combine dressing ingredients. Season to taste with salt and pepper.

Combine all salad ingredients in a large bowl and pour over dressing. Toss until ingredients are combined and fully coated in dressing. Refrigerate until ready to serve.

DINNER

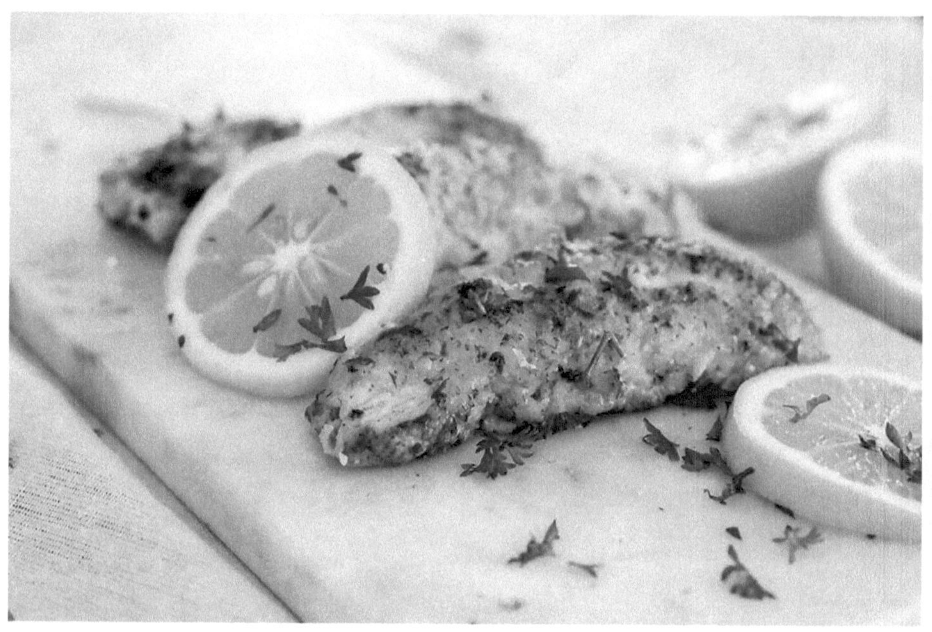

INGREDIENTS

7 ounces (200-grams) fresh Gurnard fish fillets

3 tablespoons butter

1 tablespoon lemon juice

¼ cup (25 g) fine almond flour

1 teaspoon dried dill

1 teaspoon dried chives

1 teaspoon onion powder

½ teaspoon garlic powder

Salt and pepper to taste

INSTRUCTIONS

On a large dinner plate mix together the almond flour, dill, chives, onion powder, garlic powder, salt, and pepper then spread evenly.

Take the fresh fish fillets, one at a time, and press into the flour mix. Turn and repeat. You want to really cover them well and place on a separate plate once done. You can do this in advance and hold in the fridge until cooking.

In a large pan, heat half the butter and half the lemon juice over a medium-high heat. You want it hot enough to crust the flour mix but we don't want to burn the butter or turn the juice bitter.

Let the fish cook for approximately 3 minutes. Give the pan a wriggle so the fish soaks up all the lemony butter. Don't let your pan dry out. Add more butter or lemon juice if necessary.

Place the other half of the butter and remaining lemon juice into the pan and flip the fish to cook for another 3 minutes. Again, give the pan and fish a bit of a swirl around. The coating should be nice and golden brown and you should be able to see the fish cooking through.

Check if the fish is done with a fork and remove from the pan when almost done. The fish will continue to cook so we want to avoid over cooking. If you have steamed vegetables waiting pour the butter with all the crunchy bits from the coating onto your veges. It makes a lovely dressing.

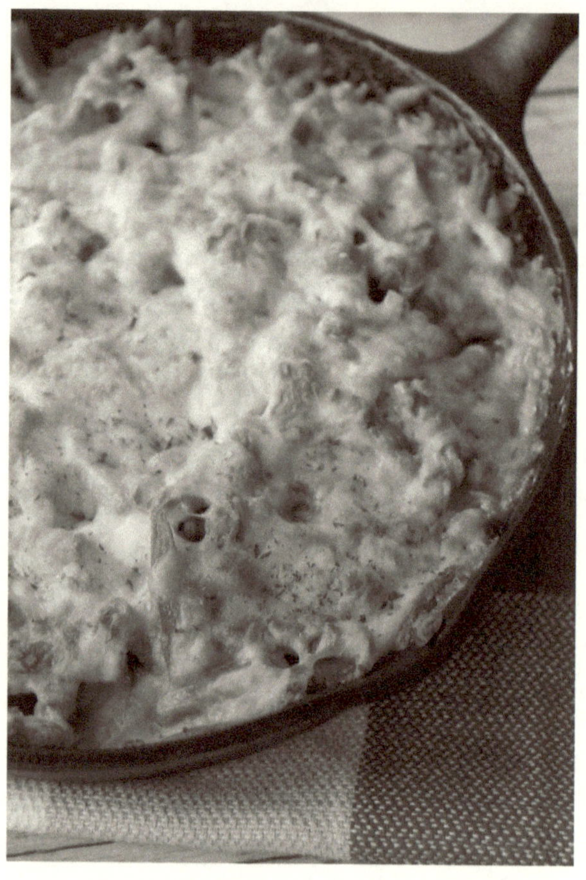

INGREDIENTS

1 pound ground beef

3 ounces cream cheese

1/2 cup beef broth

1/2 cup heavy whipping cream

2 tsp Bragg's Aminos

1 teaspoon garlic powder

2 cans green beans, drained

3/4 cup cheddar cheese

3/4 cup mozzarella cheese

1/2 teaspoon salt

1/2 teaspoon pepper

INSTRUCTIONS

Preheat oven to 350 degrees.

Brown ground beef in a cast-iron skillet then drain the excess grease.

Add cream cheese and stir until melted then add beef broth, heavy whipping cream, Bragg's Aminos, garlic powder, and salt/pepper.

Bring to a boil and cook on medium heat until mixture begins to thicken then reduce heat and simmer.

Once the ground beef mixture thickens add the two cans of green beans that have been drained on top then sprinkle cheese on top of green beans.

Bake for 25 minutes.

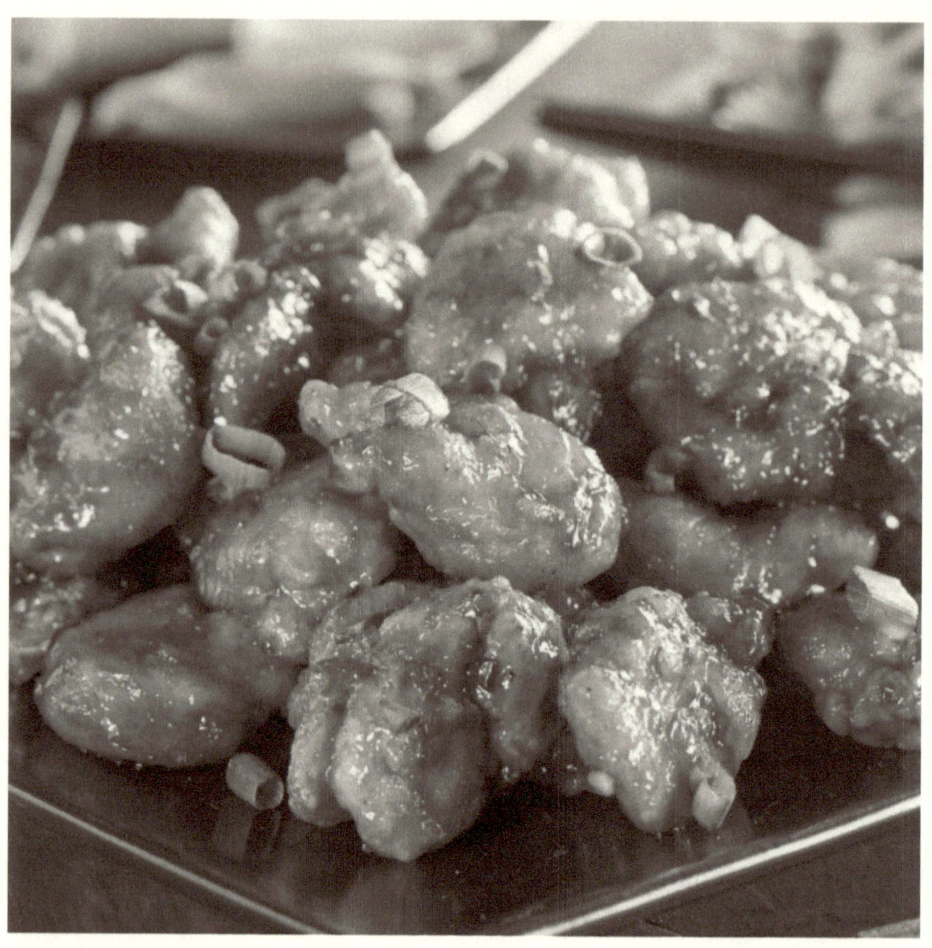

INGREDIENTS

1.5 lb boneless chicken breast halves

1/2 cup Onion, medium, chopped

2 tbsp Oilive Oil

1 tsp Salt

1 tsp Pumpkin pie spice

1 can Orange juice, frozen

2 tsp Orange zest, grated

3 cups Cranberries

1/2 cup Granular Splenda

INSTRUCTIONS

Brown chicken and onion in oil and salt in skillet over med-high heat. Add remaining ingredients, reduce heat to simmer and cook 30 minutes. Serve with hot cooked rice.

Crockpot: Add browned chicken, onions and other ingredients to crockpot.

Cook 4 hours on high or 8 hours on low

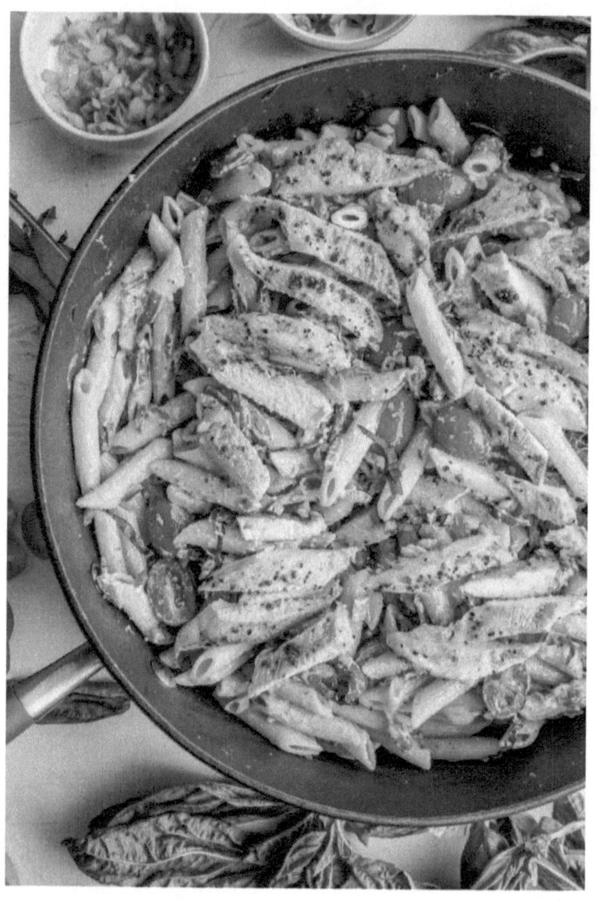

INGREDIENTS

1 pkg. (16 oz.) penne noodles, I use Dreamfields

12 oz grilled chicken breast strips, precooked (optional)

1 Tbsp. olive oil

1 cup yellow onion, diced

1 tsp. minced garlic, about 2 cloves

1/4 tsp. red pepper flakes, optional

1 large tomato, diced

1 bag baby spinach, optional

10 oz. sun dried tomato pesto sauce, (can also use basil pesto)

INSTRUCTIONS

Cook the noodles according to the package directions until they are al dente and drain them. Add spinach for the last minute of cooking.

Heat the oil in a heavy skillet over medium heat. Add the onions, garlic and red pepper flakes and sauté them until the onions are translucent, about 5 minutes. Add the tomatoes and sauté them for about 2 minutes until they soften, but don't get too mushy. Remove the onions and tomatoes from the heat.

Toss the noodles with the pesto sauce and the onion and tomato mixture and serve it immediately.

Alternatively, you can refrigerate it for up to 1 day and serve it warm or at room temperature.

Curried Turkey Burgers with Baby Spinach and Chickpea Salad

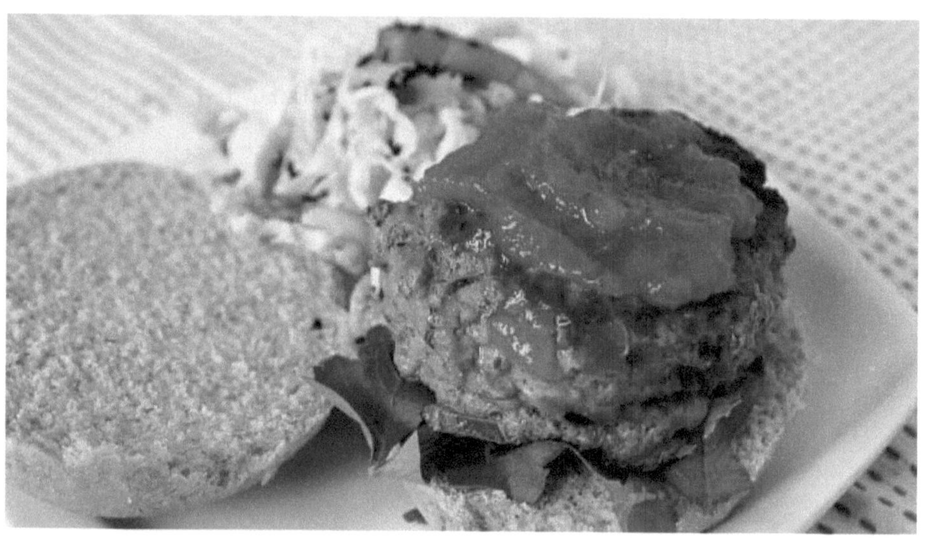

INGREDIENTS

12 ounces ground turkey

2 scallions, diagonally sliced

2 1/2 tablespoons cilantro, rinsed, patted dry, chopped

1 tablespoon ginger, grated or minced

1 tablespoon chopped garlic, jar or fresh

1 teaspoon cumin

1/2 red bell pepper, chopped

2 tablespoons Patak's mild or hot curry paste. Substitute 2 tablespoons curry powder mixed with 1 tablespoon of plain yogurt

Olive oil spray

For dessert 1/2 apple or 1 plum

1 10-ounce bag baby spinach

INSTRUCTIONS

In a mixing bowl place first eight ingredients. Combine and form into four patties. Spray burgers with olive oil. Sauté burgers in a nonstick skillet over medium high heat until cooked throughout. Serve with side of curry sauce (store bought). Accompany with the Baby Spinach and Chickpea Salad.

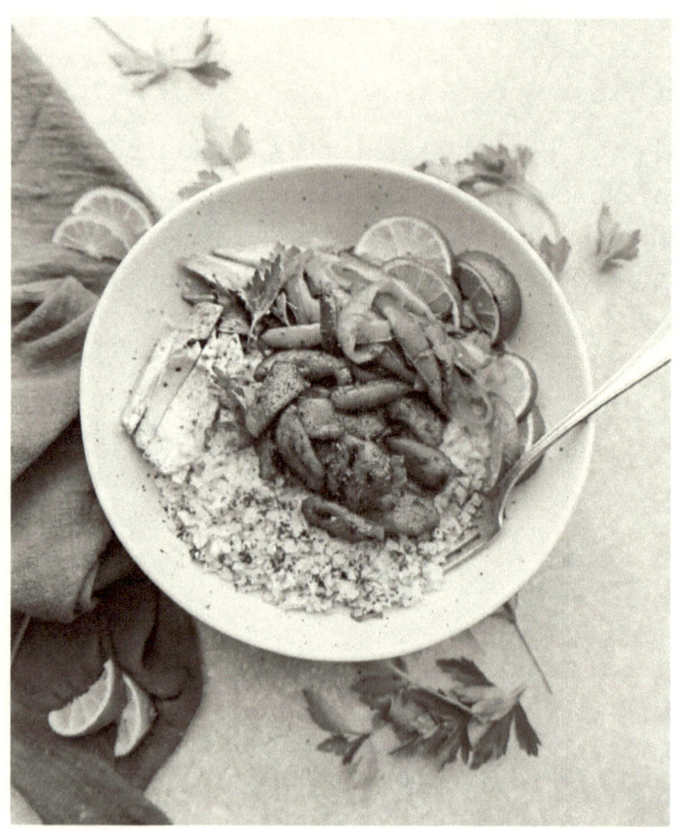

INGREDIENTS

4 ounces boneless chicken breast

2 tablespoons salsa

2 tablespoons bottled lime juice

Salt to taste

Freshly ground black pepper to taste

1/4 cup water or more

1/3 green pepper, cut into quarters, seeds and membrane removed

1/3 red pepper, cut into quarters, seeds and membrane removed

1/3 yellow onion, sliced into 1/4-inch-wide rings, and microwaved
on high for 2 minutes, stirring after 1 minute

1   fajita-size (8-inch) tortilla

1/2 cup chopped tomato

4 tablespoons guacamole

1/2 cup strawberries

INSTRUCTIONS

Slice chicken breasts crosswise into 1/2-inch strips. Place in a glass
dish with salsa, lime juice, salt, and pepper and enough water to cover.
Cover with plastic wrap and refrigerate overnight. Into a large skillet,
over high heat, pour in the liquid from the chicken and cook to reduce
by half. Add the chicken strips and using a wide wooden spatula, toss
frequently. When chicken turns opaque but is not yet thoroughly
cooked, add the peppers and onion. Continue cooking and tossing the
mixture. Cook until the liquid has evaporated and it begins to sizzle.
Give one more toss and remove from heat. Serve with tortilla and
condiments. Serve strawberries for dessert.

Mex-Chicken Chili (Burritos)

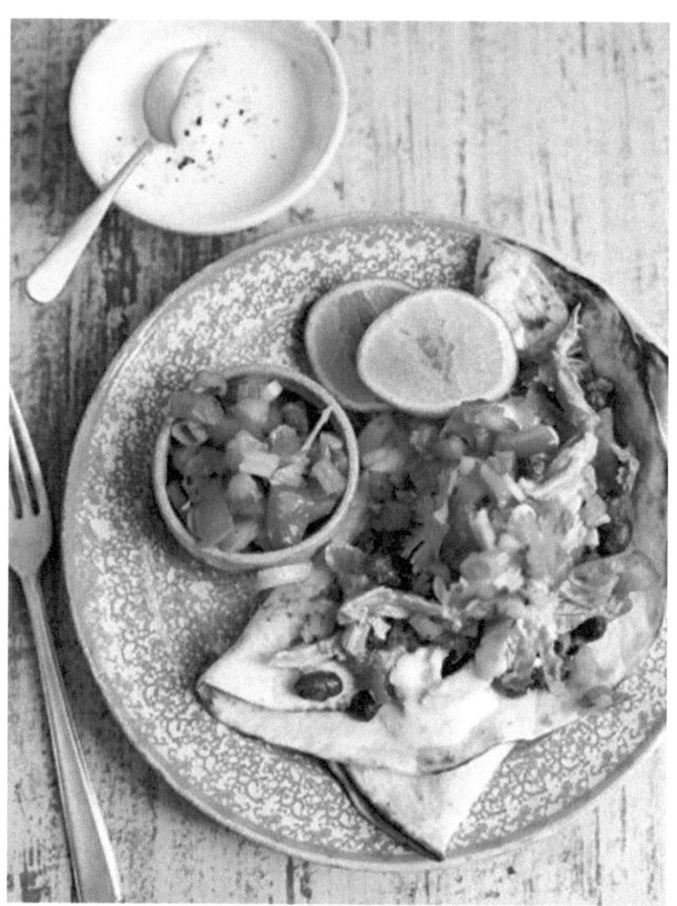

INGREDIENTS

3 ounces cooked chicken, cut into one-inch cubes

1 ounce low-fat shredded cheese

1/2 cup no-salt added cooked, drained black beans

1/2 cup salsa

12 black olives, chopped

Chili powder and/or cayenne pepper to taste

1/2 orange sliced

INSTRUCTIONS

Combine all the ingredients, except the orange into a microwave-safe
bowl and mix. Microwave until hot and serve.

Beef Italiano

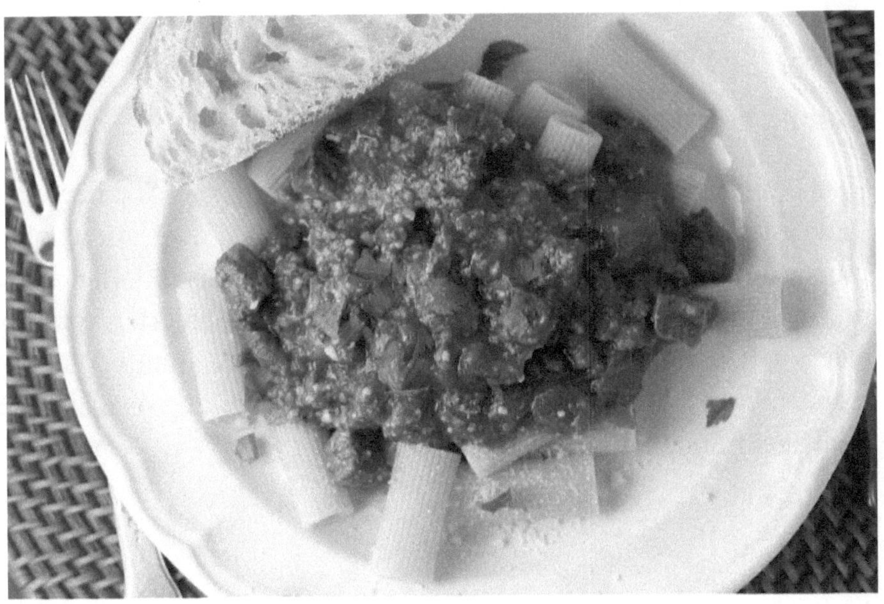

INGREDIENTS

4 ounces lean beef, small cubes

1/2 cup Zoned Italian Sauce

1 cup Italian-style green beans

2 cups red and green pepper strips

3/4 cup onion, diced

1/4 cup salsa

1 1/3 teaspoons olive oil, divided

1/2 teaspoon parsley flakes

1/2 teaspoon Worcestershire sauce

1/2 teaspoon celery salt

1/8 teaspoon lemon herb seasoning

1/8 teaspoon dried oregano

INSTRUCTIONS

Heat 2/3 teaspoon oil in a medium nonstick sauté pan. Add beef and sauté until cooked. Add Zoned Italian Sauce and simmer for 3 to 5 minutes. In second nonstick sauté pan, heat remaining oil. Sauté the green beans, pepper strips, onion, salsa, parsley, Worcestershire sauce, celery salt, lemon herb seasoning, and oregano. Cook until crisp-tender, about 5 minutes. Spoon vegetables onto serving dish and top with beef mixture.

Orange Herbed Chicken Stew

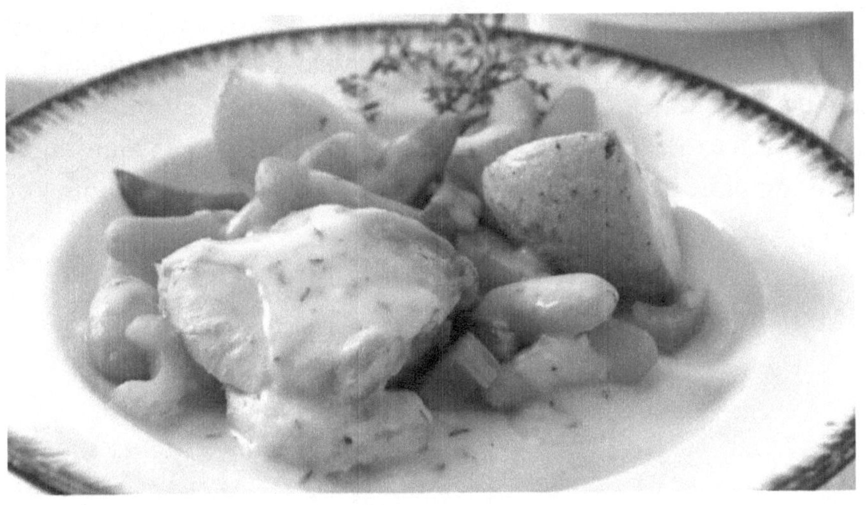

INGREDIENTS

3 ounces   chicken tenderloin, diced

1/3 cup orange juice

1/3 cup Mandarin oranges

4 cups mushrooms, sliced

1 teaspoon   olive oil, divided

1 tablespoon cider vinegar

1 tablespoon parsley, chopped

1/2 teaspoon garlic, chopped

1/2 teaspoon pure orange extract

Salt and pepper, to taste

INSTRUCTIONS

In a medium nonstick sauté pan, heat 2/3 teaspoon oil. Add chicken, vinegar, parsley, garlic, and salt and pepper. In a second nonstick sauté pan heat remaining oil and sauté mushrooms until they soften. Add orange juice, oranges, and orange extract to the first pan and simmer for 3 minutes. Place mushrooms in a serving bowl and top with chicken mixture.

Fish in Green Olive Sauce

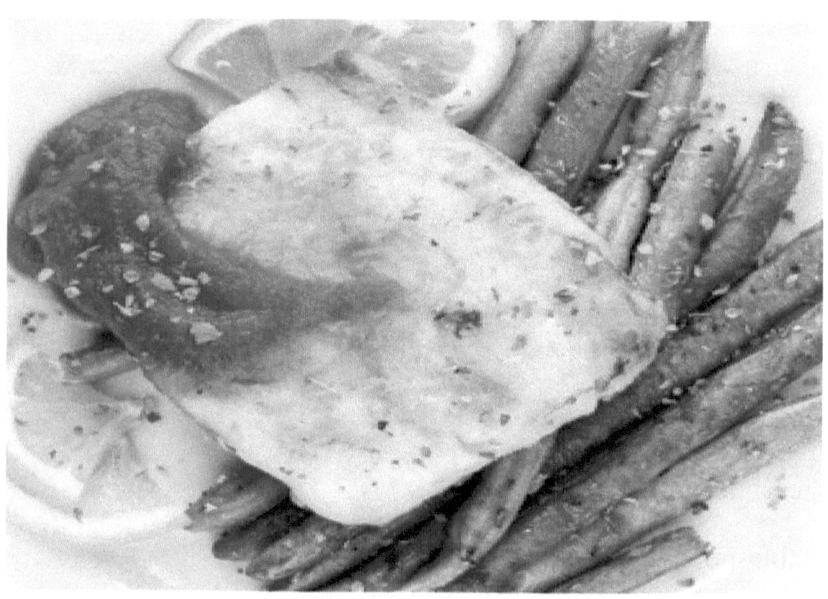

INGREDIENTS

4 ½ oz. cod or haddock

1 teaspoon olive oil

1 cup   onion chopped

1 cup   tomato chopped

1   green pepper chopped

¼ cup slice green olives

1 Tablespoon capers

1 Tablespoon parsley

1 Tablespoon cilantro

1 teaspoon wine vinegar

1 cup mixed berries or 1 apple or 1 orange or 1 pear

INSTRUCTIONS

Heat the olive oil in an oven proof sauté pan over medium heat. Add in onion, green pepper and sauté for 2 minutes. Add in green olives, capers, parsley, cilantro and wine vinegar cook for another 2-3 minutes. Add the fish and place in the oven at 325 degrees until fish is flaky, about 12-15 minutes. Have fruit for dessert.

SNACKS

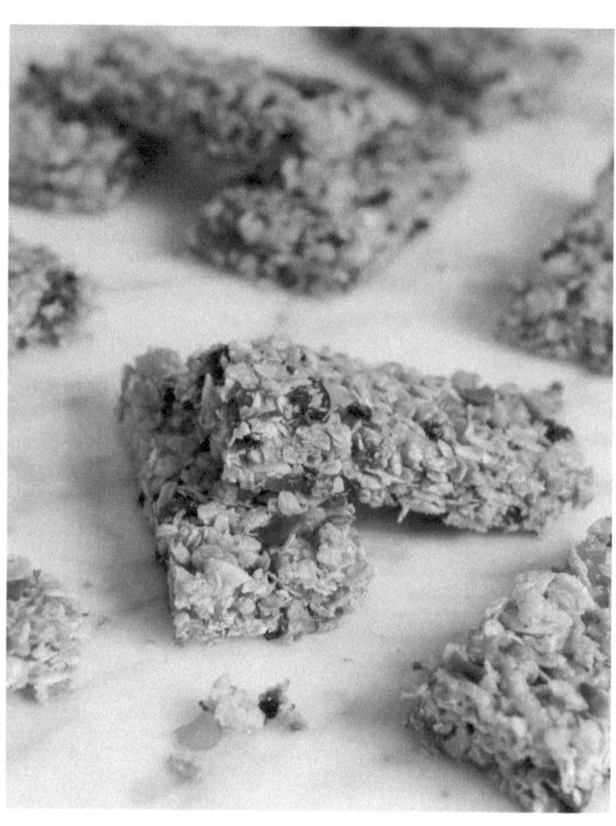

INGREDIENTS

210 grams large flake oats

3 cups water

100 grams raisins

120 grams soy protein powder

4 egg whites

1 cup soya milk, (unsweetened)

3.25 tablespoons olive oil

1/2 teaspoon baking soda

1/2 teaspoon cinnamon

5 tablespoons Fry's Cocoa

5-10 drops liquid Stevia

INSTRUCTIONS

Mix oats into 3 cups of boiling water. Lower the heat to medium and stir for 10 minutes. Spread on a cookie sheet and leave to dry for 30 minutes. After 15 minutes cut into 8 rectangles and flip over for the second 15 minutes.

Mix egg whites, 3 tablespoons of olive oil, liquid Stevia and soya milk in a bowl.

Mix the protein powder, cocoa, raisins, baking soda and cinnamon in a separate bowl.

Mix the liquid and dry ingredients together thoroughly.

Mix in the cooked oats one chunk at a time and thoroughly mix. Lightly grease the bottom of the baking dish with a bit of olive oil.

 Put half in an 8-by-8-inch baking dish and bake at 375 F for 25 to 30 minutes. Cut into 6 equal rectangles and put on a plate to cool. Repeat with other half.

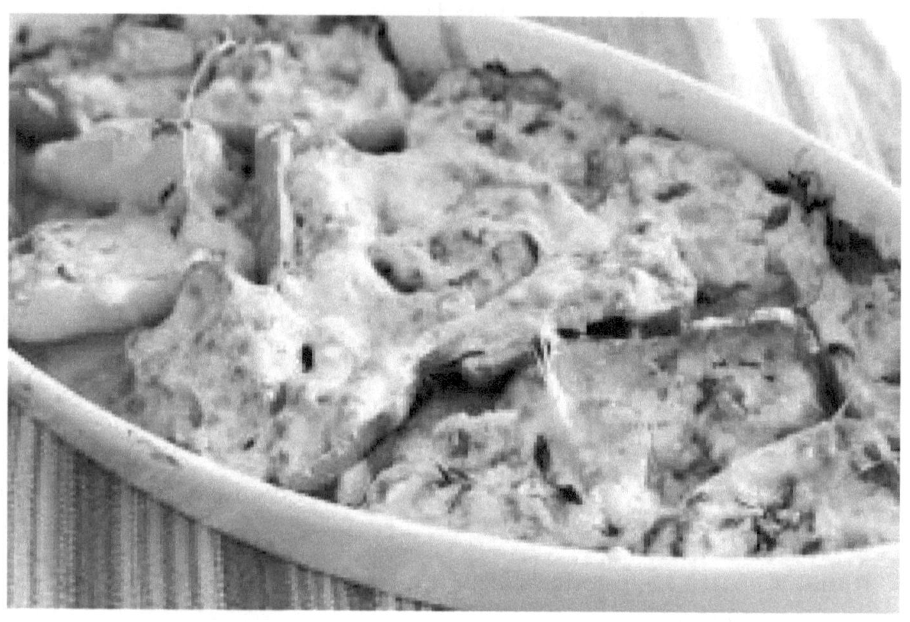

INGREDIENTS

- 8 oz. mini bell peppers, about 2 per serving

- 1 oz. air-dried chorizo, finely chopped

- 1 tbsp fresh thyme, finely chopped or fresh cilantro

- 8 oz. cream cheese

- ½ tbsp mild chipotle paste

- 2 tbsp olive oil

- 4 oz. shredded cheese

INSTRUCTIONS

Set the oven to 325°F (200°C). Split the bell peppers lengthwise and remove the core.

Finely chop the chorizo and the herbs.

Mix together the cream cheese, spices and oil in a small bowl. Add the chorizo and herbs. Stir until smooth.

Fill the bell peppers with the mixture and place in a greased baking dish.

Sprinkle shredded cheese on top.

Bake in the oven for 15–20 minutes or until the cheese is melted and golden brown.

Salad sandwiches

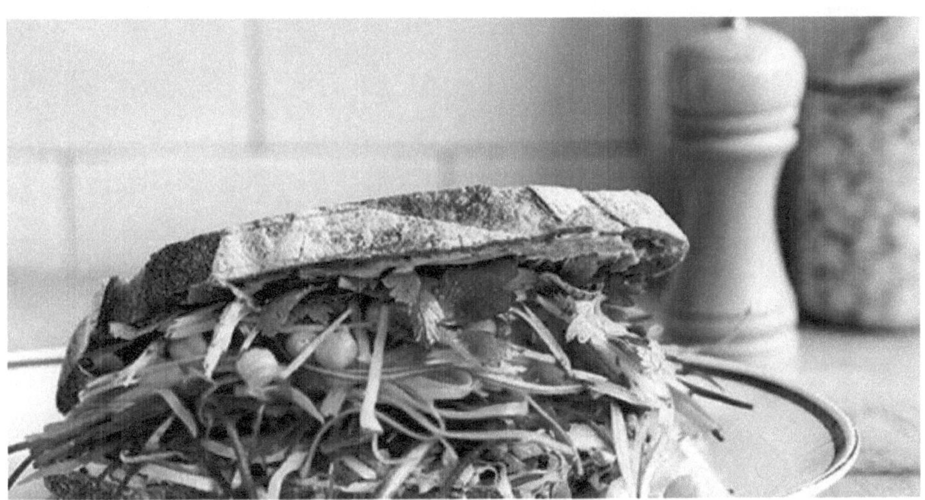

INGREDIENTS

2 oz. Romaine lettuce or baby gem lettuce

½ oz. butter

1 oz. edam cheese or other cheese of your liking

½ avocado

1 cherry tomatoes

INSTRUCTIONS

Rinse the lettuce thoroughly and use as a base for the toppings.

Smear butter on the lettuce leaves and slice the cheese, avocado and tomato and add on top.

Low-carb cream cheese with herbs

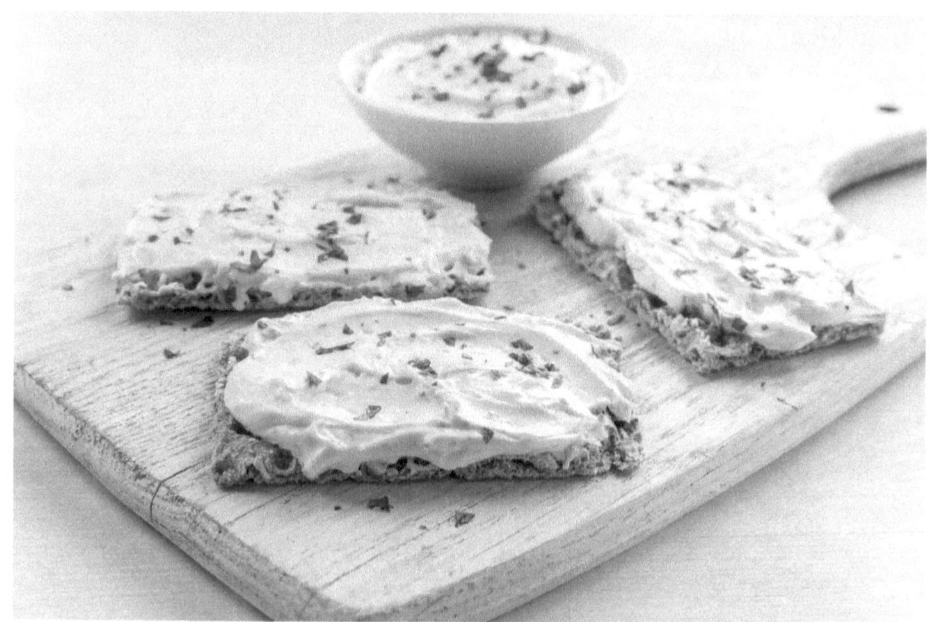

INGREDIENTS

8 oz. cream cheese

2 tsp olive oil

½ cup fresh parsley or fresh basil, chopped

1 garlic clove, minced

1 tsp lemon zest

salt and pepper, to taste

4 celery stalks, or other fresh vegetables of your liking

INSTRUCTIONS

Stir all ingredients into the cream cheese. Let sit in the refrigerator for at least 10 minutes to let all the flavors develop. Add salt if needed.

Rinse celery stalks, cut into 2-3 inch lengths, and serve together with the soft cheese.

Caprese snack

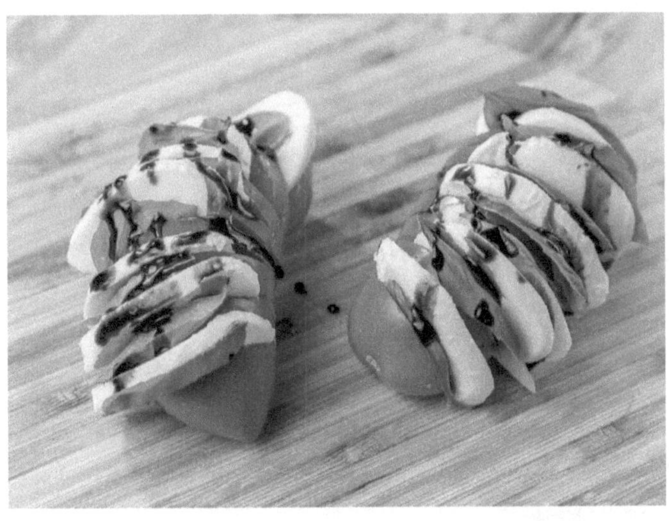

INGREDIENTS

8 oz. cherry tomatoes

8 oz. mozzarella, mini cheese balls

2 tbsp green pesto

salt and pepper

INSTRUCTIONS

Cut the tomatoes and mozzarella balls in half. Add pesto and stir.

Salt and pepper to taste.

Low-carb sesame crispbread

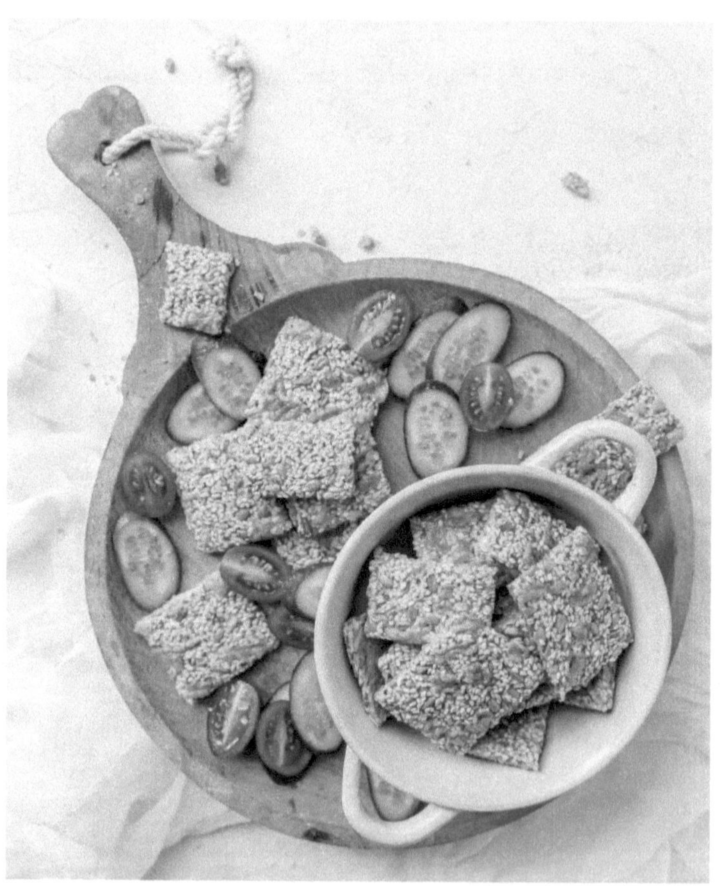

INGREDIENTS

1¼ cups sesame seeds

½ cup sunflower seeds

2 oz. shredded cheese, like Gouda or cheddar

1 tbsp ground psyllium husk powder

½ cup water

2 eggs

¼ tsp salt

INSTRUCTIONS

Preheat the oven to 350°F (175°C). Line a 13"x18" (33x46 cm) baking sheet with parchment paper.

Add all of the ingredients to a medium-sized bowl and stir to combine. Spread the mixture (about 1/8" thick or 3.1 mm) onto the parchment paper, sprinkle with sea salt, and bake for 20 minutes.

Remove the crispbread from the oven, and carefully cut into desired form.

Lower the heat to 275°F (135°C) and put the crispbread back into the oven for another 30-40 minutes, or until lightly golden in color.

Check the crispbread to make sure it is completely dry without any moist areas. Keep it in the oven with the door slightly open, until the oven is cool.

Keto garlic bread

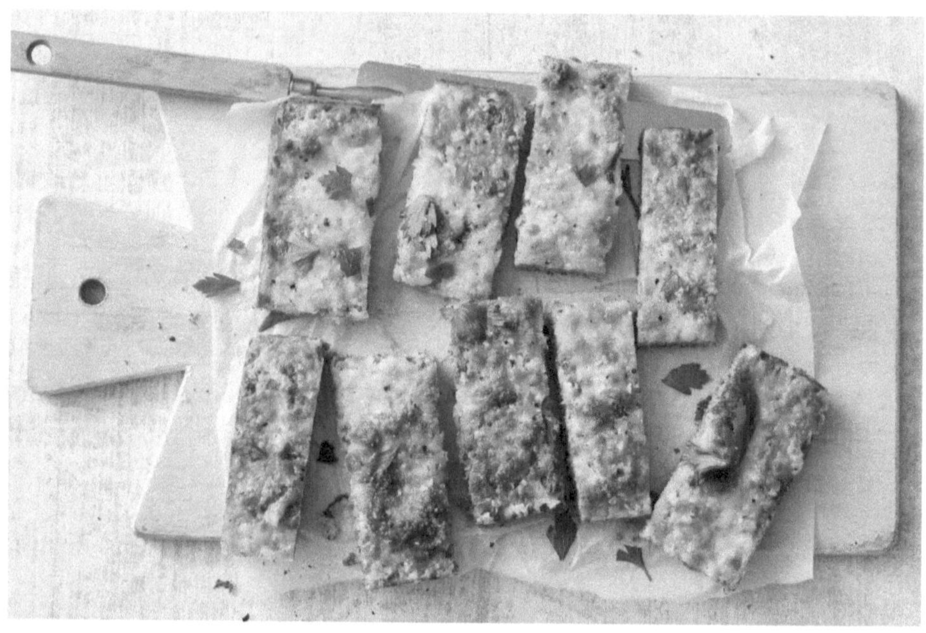

INGREDIENTS

Bread

- 1¼ cups almond flour

- 5 tbsp ground psyllium husk powder

- 2 tsp baking powder

- 1 tsp sea salt

- 2 tsp cider vinegar or white wine vinegar

- 1 cup boiling water

- 3 egg whites

Garlic butter

4 oz. butter, at room temperature

1 garlic clove, minced

2 tbsp fresh parsley, finely chopped

½ tsp salt

INSTRUCTIONS

Preheat the oven to 350°F (175°C). Mix the dry ingredients for the bread in a bowl.

Bring the water to a boil and add this, the vinegar and egg whites to the bowl, while whisking with a hand mixer for about 30 seconds. Don't overmix the dough, the consistency should resemble Play-Doh.

Form with moist hands into 10 pieces and roll into hot dog buns. Make sure to leave enough space between them on the baking sheet to double in size.

Bake on lower rack in oven for 40-50 minutes, they're done when you can hear a hollow sound when tapping the bottom of the bun.

Make the garlic butter while the bread is baking. Mix all the ingredients together and put in the fridge.

Take the buns out of the oven when they're done and leave to let cool. Take the garlic butter out of the fridge. When the buns are cooled, cut them in halves, using a serrated knife, and spread garlic butter on each half.

Turn your oven up to 425°F (225°C) and bake the garlic bread for 10-15 minutes, until golden brown.

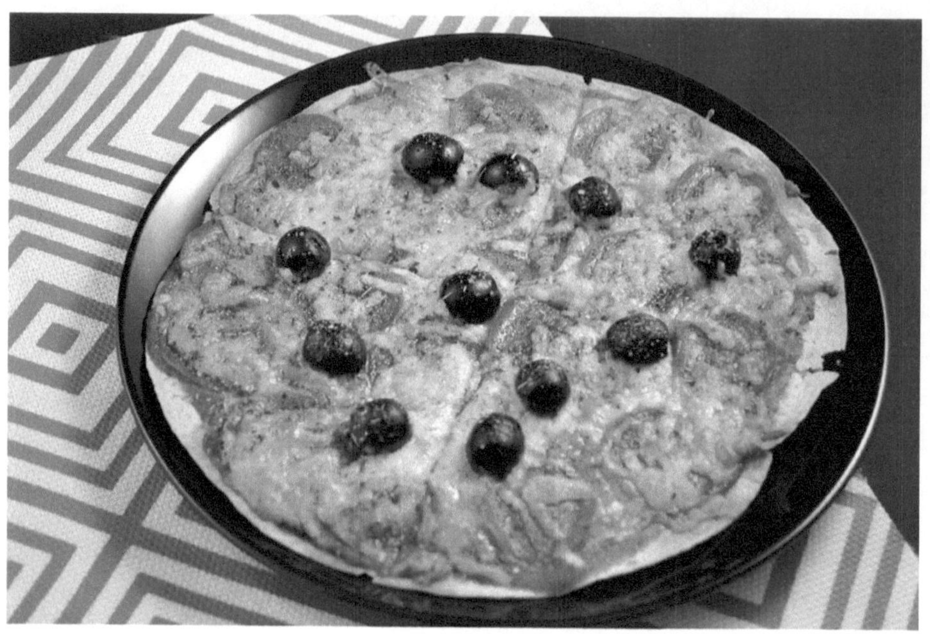

INGREDIENTS

Topping

½ cup unsweetened tomato sauce

8 oz. shredded cheese

2 tsp dried basil or dried oregano

salt and pepper (optional)

Low-carb tortillas

2 eggs

2 egg whites

6 oz. cream cheese

¼ tsp salt

1 tsp ground psyllium husk powder

1 tbsp coconut flour

INSTRUCTIONS

Tortillas

Preheat the oven to 400°F (200°C).

Whisk the eggs and egg whites fluffy and continue to whisk with a hand mixer, preferably for a few minutes. Add cream cheese and continue to whisk until the batter is smooth.

Mix salt, psyllium husk and coconut flour in a small bowl. Add the flour mix one spoon at a time into the batter and continue to whisk some more. Let the batter sit for a few minutes, or until the batter is thick like an American pancake batter. How fast the batter will swell depends on the brand of psyllium husk – some trial and error might be needed.

Bring out two baking sheets and place parchment paper on each. Using a spatula, spread the batter thinly (no more than ¼ inch thick) into 4–6 circles or 2 rectangles.

Bake on upper rack for about 5 minutes or more, until the tortilla turns a little brown around the edges. Carefully check the bottom side so that it doesn't burn.

Pizza

Turn your oven up to 450°F (225°C).

Spread 1-2 tablespoons of tomato paste, sauce or ajvar (roasted red pepper sauce) on each low-carb tortilla bread. Salt and pepper if needed.

Bake the mini pizzas in the oven until the cheese has melted.

Stuffed mini bell peppers

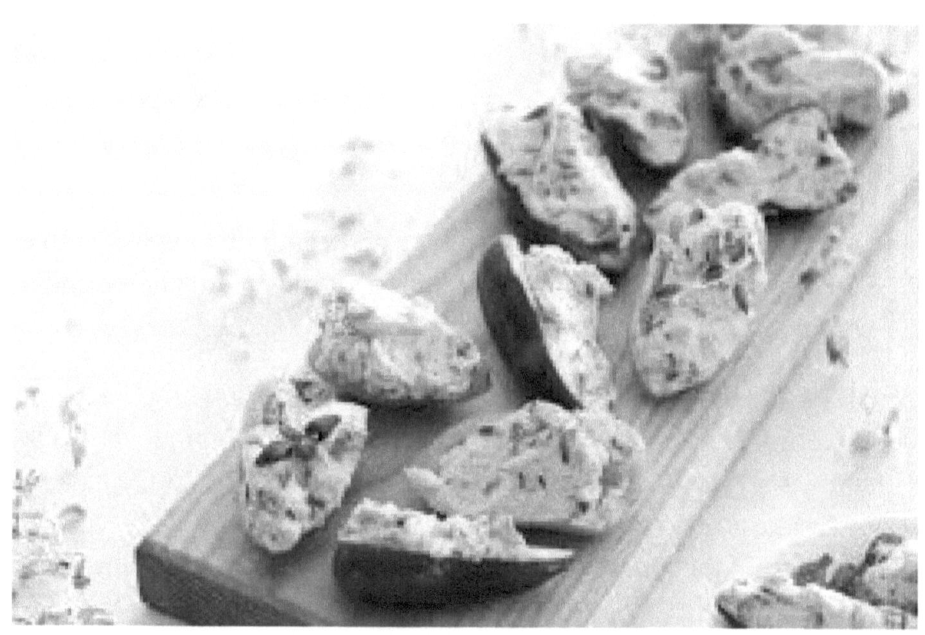

INGREDIENTS

8 mini bell peppers

8 oz. cream cheese

1 oz. air-dried chorizo, thinly sliced

½ tbsp mild chipotle paste

2 tbsp olive oil

1 tbsp fresh thyme or fresh cilantro

INSTRUCTIONS

Split the bell peppers lengthwise and remove the core.

Chop the sausage and herbs finely.

Mix cheese, spices and oil in a small bowl. Add sausage and herbs, and stir together.

Spread out the cheese cream into the bell peppers and serve as a snack or appetizer.

Keto egg muffins

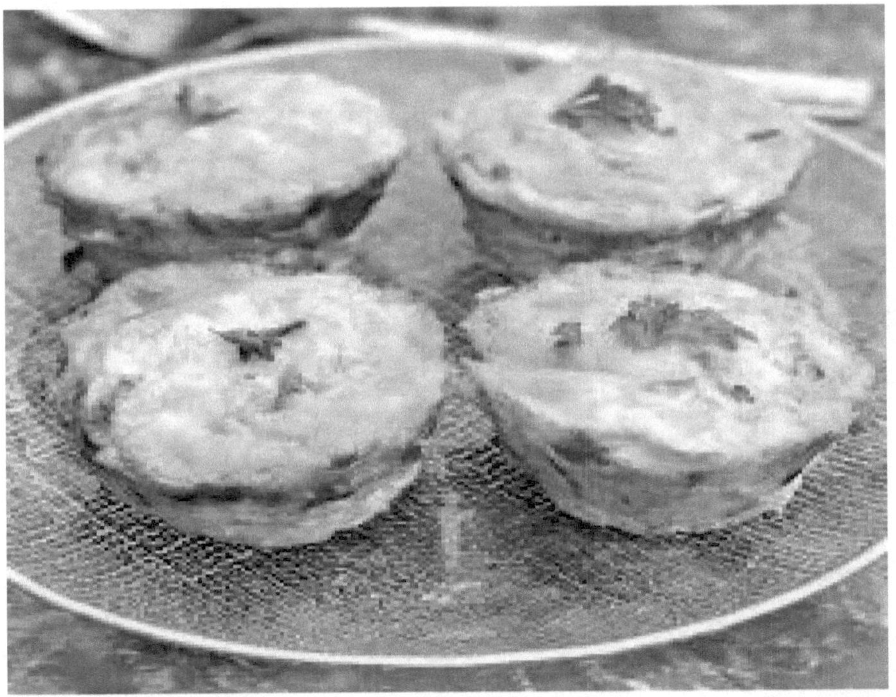

INGREDIENTS

2 scallions, finely chopped

5 oz. chopped air-dried chorizo or salami or cooked bacon

12 eggs

2 tbsp red pesto or green pesto (optional)

salt and pepper

6 oz. shredded cheese

INSTRUCTIONS

Preheat the oven to 350°F (175°C).

Line a muffin tin with non-stick, insertable baking cups or grease a silicone muffin tin with butter.

Add scallions and chorizo to the bottom of the tin.

Whisk eggs together with pesto, salt and pepper. Add the cheese and stir.

Pour the batter on top of the scallions and chorizo.

Bake for 15–20 minutes, depending on the size of the muffin tin.